Understanding Addiction

Belinda Tobin

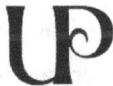

UP

UNDERSTANDING PRESS

Understanding Addiction

Copyright © 2024 by Belinda Tobin

Published by Understanding Press

UP

Paperback ISBN: 978-1-7637062-2-4

E-Book ISBN - 978-1-7637062-3-1

For permissions or enquiries, please contact:

Understanding Press

Email: up@heart-led.pub

Website: www.heart-led.pub/understanding-press

First Edition: October 2024

NATIONAL LIBRARY OF AUSTRALIA — A catalogue record for this book is available from the National Library of Australia

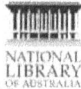

Other titles in The Understanding Series:

Understanding Violence

Understanding Sexuality

Understanding Monogamy

Understanding Creativity

I acknowledge the Yuggera and Ugarapul peoples as the Traditional Owners of the lands and waterways where this book was written. I honour the wisdom that lives within the cultures of our First Nations peoples and celebrate its continuity. I pay my deep respects to Elders past, present and future and send my greatest gratitude for all they do for the life of this land.

Always was, always will be.

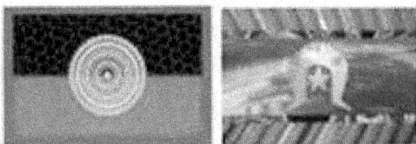

Contents

Section 5 - Connecting With Spirit

Section 6 - Creating a Supportive Environment

Section 7 - Key Challenges in Healing from Addiction

Section 8 - Essential Skills

An Important Note

This book has been written as a source of information and inspiration, but it should not be taken as medical advice.

Always seek the guidance of your doctor or other qualified health professional with any questions regarding your general health or a specific medical condition. Their expertise and personalised advice are crucial for your wellbeing.

Never disregard the advice of a medical professional, or delay seeking it, because of something you have read in this book.

If you are struggling with an addiction, or have a loved one who is, please reach out for help. Seeking help is not a sign of weakness—it is the strongest thing you can do. Your bravery could be the change needed to break generations of harm.

A list of organisations you can contact immediately is provided at the back of this book. They are ready to take your call.

Introduction

One of the most traumatic times of my life was when I stood up in an Alcoholics Anonymous meeting and said:

"Hi, I'm Belinda, and I am an addict."

While yes, there was an initial sense of relief at admitting the truth, at the same time, it was like all the shame, guilt, fear, and anger I felt came tumbling down upon me. Instead of being liberated by the admission, I was suffocated by my distress. Hearing repeatedly about what other people had lost added more rubble on top of my hurting heart, and there was no doubt about it: I was trapped in a deep, dark cave.

It has taken me many years to crawl out of what felt like a hopeless prison and see the light. Thanks to some very patient loved ones and some insightful and compassionate guides, I have learnt so much through this process. This book is here to share this knowledge with you, for understanding gives us the power to take wise and effective action. It also gives us the chance to come to a place of deep and true love for ourselves and for others.

"Understanding is love's other name. If you don't understand, you can't love." ~ Thich Nhat Hahn

My research and reflections have resulted in a model of addiction called The Addiction Healing Pathway. This model explains the fundamental cause of addiction, its flow-on effects, and, more importantly, the process of healing. However, it is not just a model based on my ideas. It comes from a combination of ancient wisdom, such as spiritual teachings and philosophies, and modern science, including neurobiology and psychology. It shows how we need both approaches to deal with the disease of addiction at its source.

As you will see, the Addiction Healing Pathway's fundamental premise is that it is the separation from our unique and life-sustaining spirits that causes addiction. This disconnect creates an internal conflict that fuels distressing emotions, harmful thoughts, beliefs and behaviours. What begins as a spiritual crisis ends as a war on the body and mind, and there are many casualties. Throughout the pages of this book, this pathway will be presented. I hope that it may help you understand what causes people to undertake such extreme self-harm, but also the steps required to move towards a place of healing and hope.

Throughout *Understanding Addiction*, you will notice that I use the word healing instead of recovery. I know for some, the difference may be minimal. Still, for me, it is an important distinction to make. I have chosen healing instead of recovery because I believe you never really 'recover' from addiction. It is not just something you get over, like a chest infection, and then move on with life. The wounds go deep. Like soldiers never forget the harrows of war, I don't think someone with an addiction can ever recapture the person they once were. They have seen too much, felt and caused too much pain to 'get back to normal'. Besides, as you will see, it is likely that trying to be 'normal' caused so much of the suffering in the first place.

The one thing I have learnt from my experience is that the horror of addiction never leaves. But you do have a choice - to let the shame suck you down into the dark and keep you stuck or to find the courage to show yourself compassion. We can care for the wounds, nurse the scars and use the wisdom we have gained to help others.

For those of you who are suffering from addiction or are caring for someone who is, please remember:

You deserve to lead a healthy and happy life. Let this book be your guide.

Section 1- Understanding the Cause of Addiction

More Advancement = More Addiction

"Technological progress has merely provided us with more efficient means for going backwards." ~ *Aldous Huxley*

Addiction is a growing global concern, affecting millions of individuals across various demographics. According to the World Health Organization (WHO), 283 million people worldwide suffer from alcohol use disorder, and 1.3 billion are addicted to tobacco. Additionally, 35 million people are affected by drug use disorders, with approximately ten million individuals seeking assistance for gambling addiction in the last year alone[1].

Expanding Scope of Addictions

Recent trends indicate that the range of addictive behaviours is broadening beyond traditional substances. In 2017, it was estimated that 18 million people, or more than six per cent of those aged 12 and older, misused prescription medications, including opioids, sedatives, and stimulants[2]. Furthermore, emerging reports highlight increasing addictions to behaviours such as excessive eating and compulsive sexual activity.

Recent studies reveal that eating addictions, including binge eating disorder, are on the rise globally. This type of addiction often manifests as a compulsive need to consume large amounts of food despite negative consequences, such as obesity, diabetes, and cardiovascular disease. In the United

States alone, it is estimated that around 2.8 per cent of adults experience binge eating disorder during their lifetime. This prevalence underscores the significant mental and physical health impacts, with many cases co-occurring with other addictions, such as alcoholism or substance abuse, highlighting the intertwined nature of behavioural and chemical dependencies.

Restrictive eating disorders, such as anorexia nervosa, can also be understood through the lens of addiction, where individuals develop a compulsive need to control and restrict their food intake. Anorexia nervosa affects approximately 0.9 per cent of women and 0.3 per cent of men in their lifetime. A global study revealed that the prevalence of eating disorders increased significantly over the last three decades, with adolescent populations being particularly affected. In Australia, recent estimates suggest that up to 12 per cent of adolescents aged 15 to 19 experienced an eating disorder in 2023, reflecting an upward trend in diagnoses within this age group.

Cosmetic surgery addiction, also known as body dysmorphic disorder-related addiction, is a growing concern as procedures become more accessible and normalized. This condition often involves an obsessive need for physical alterations, despite prior surgeries, fueled by dissatisfaction with appearance and underlying mental health issues like anxiety or low self-esteem. Statistics on addiction to cosmetic surgery are challenging to quantify precisely, as this behavior often stems from conditions like body dysmorphic disorder (BDD). However, it is estimated that between 4% and 15% of individuals seeking cosmetic surgery may suffer from BDD, a condition strongly linked to an obsessive desire for repeated surgical procedures.

Similarly, sex and pornography addictions are becoming increasingly recognized as pervasive issues in the modern era. Studies estimate that 3-6 per cent of the population may struggle with compulsive sexual behavior, with a significant proportion of these cases involving addiction to pornography. In 2021, one survey suggested that 10-15 per cent of internet users frequent pornographic websites regularly, with some developing patterns of dependency that disrupt personal relationships, professional life, and mental health. These figures reveal a growing need for awareness and resources to address the broader scope of behavioural addictions.

In 2019, the WHO recognised gaming disorder as an official addiction, reflecting the growing concern over behavioural addictions. In response, several countries, including the United Kingdom and the United States, established clinics dedicated to treating internet addiction. In the United States alone, it is estimated that eight per cent of the population, or over 26 million people, are addicted to the internet, struggling to balance real-world activities with online interactions such as social media, internet shopping, and gaming.

There is also a concerning trend in the decreasing age of individuals affected by internet addiction. In South Korea, at least 160,000 children aged five to nine are reported to be addicted to the Internet. In Japan, approximately 500,000 children aged 12 to 18 meet the criteria for internet addiction. Similarly, in China, about ten per cent of teenagers, equating to 14.5 million individuals, are classified as internet addicts[3].

The rise of vaping and e-cigarettes represents a new frontier in addictive behaviours, especially for adolescents. It is estimated that there are over 55 million vape users globally, with a significant proportion being teenagers. The National Institute on Drug Abuse notes that one-third of these users transition to traditional tobacco products within six months, a phenomenon known as the 'gateway effect', which highlights the potential risks associated with vaping. No longer are vapes seen as an effective way to help smokers quit the toxic substances within cigarettes. They have now become a source of self-harm within themselves.

Defining Addiction

Traditionally, addiction has been narrowly defined as physical and mental dependence on a substance[4]. However, the evolving landscape of addictions demands a more comprehensive definition. It's no longer just about substances like alcohol, tobacco, opioids, and illicit drugs. It's also about everyday activities like eating, sexual behaviour, internet use, and even cosmetic surgery. This broader understanding of addiction is essential for a more effective approach to prevention and treatment.

Dr Gabor Maté offers a more inclusive definition of addiction:

"Any behaviour that gives you temporary relief, temporary pleasure, but in the long term causes harm, has some negative consequences, and you can't give it up, despite those negative consequences."[5]

This perspective underscores the multifaceted nature of addiction, extending beyond substance dependence to include behavioural patterns that provide temporary relief but lead to long-term detriment.

The Paradox of Progress

The proliferation of addictive behaviours raises important questions about the relationship between human advancement and addiction. As societies make strides in scientific, medical, and technological fields, there appears to be a concurrent increase in the prevalence of addiction. Everything we invent to remove pain, bring enjoyment or to make our lives easier is being twisted to become a source of powerlessness and distress. This paradox shows that current approaches to understanding and treating addiction are incomplete and that we need to dig deeper into the underlying causes of addiction. For it seems somewhere amongst all this complexity, technology, entertainment and excess, we are losing the link to an essential life-sustaining source.

Core Concepts

Addiction is a growing global issue, with millions suffering from various substance use disorders, including alcohol, tobacco, drugs, and gambling.

Beyond traditional substances, addictions now include behavioural patterns such as internet use, gaming, excessive eating, and compulsive sexual activity. This evolution reflects a need for a broader definition and understanding of addiction.

Younger populations are increasingly affected by addiction, with concerning rates of internet and vaping addiction reported among children and teenagers worldwide.

Traditional definitions of addiction, focused on substance dependence, are no longer sufficient. Modern definitions encompass a wide range of behaviours that provide temporary relief but cause long-term harm.

There is a paradox where societal advancements in technology, medicine, and entertainment coincide with increasing rates of addiction. This suggests that current approaches to understanding and treating addiction may be incomplete, pointing to a need for a deeper exploration of its underlying causes and a reconnection to essential, life-sustaining values.

Current Viewpoints on Addiction

"A lot of people think that addiction is a choice. A lot of people think it's a matter of will. That has not been my experience. I don't find it to have anything to do with strength." ~ Matthew Perry

For as long as there has been addiction, there have been people who have sought to understand it, and to develop models to drive its treatment. While working through these different theories may seem tedious, understanding the differing viewpoints is important, for they all provide part of the picture of what addiction is, and therefore, how it can be overcome. For those seeking or currently undergoing treatment, it is also helpful to recognise the perspectives held by the healthcare providers you are working with, as their beliefs about addiction will shape the treatment programs they recommend. In this way, familiarising oneself with these different approaches towards addiction can help you make informed choices about services and treatment options.

Addiction as a Choice

One viewpoint is that addiction is fundamentally a choice. Choice is defined as:

"An act of choosing between two or more possibilities"[6].

From an outsider's perspective, it may appear that individuals do have the power to choose whether or not to engage in addictive behaviours; that they have the ability to decide whether to drink, use a substance, or spend time gaming or internet shopping.

This perspective aligns with the ideas of Viktor Frankl, a psychiatrist and Holocaust survivor, who stated:

"Between the stimulus and the response is a space, and in that space is your power and your freedom."

However, as we will see in the following sections when we look at addiction as a brain disease, it becomes apparent that addictive behaviours can become hard-wired into the brain, making them automatic and subconscious. As a result, the 'space' Frankl refers to may diminish or become almost imperceptible. Yes, a person would have had a choice in the beginning of the addiction process in terms of choosing whether to take the substance or engage in the activity. But as they continued to repeat the behaviour, their ability to make good choices would have slowly been reduced. As the brain and body become dependent on the substance or behaviour the person's ability to choose alternative activities would have been severely compromised.

A vivid illustration of this is depicted in the film 'Pleasure Unwoven' by Dr Kevin McCauley[7], where an individual faces a life-threatening dilemma at a bar. If he drinks a glass of whisky, he will be shot. A rational person would naturally avoid the drink to preserve their life. However, for a person with an addiction, the compulsion to drink is so overpowering that they might risk being shot just to satisfy their craving. This example demonstrates the extent to which addiction can impair cognitive function, compromising the ability to make rational decisions[8]. In addiction, the brain's circuits that govern decision-making and self-control fail to operate normally, creating a state of immediate, desperate need.

Despite evidence that addiction impairs decision-making, the Choice Model persists, often viewing addiction as a result of personal weakness, a lack of moral fibre or simple selfishness. This perspective suggests that individuals with addictions should be held responsible for their choices, and if harm is inflicted upon others, they must be punished to enforce personal accountability.

One positive aspect of the Choice Model is that it emphasises personal power and responsibility, for these are important factors in healing. However, these aspects can only be beneficial when an individual is mentally and physically equipped to handle them constructively. It is unreasonable to expect someone whose decision-making abilities have been compromised by addiction to immediately make sound choices. The emphasis on choice is vital to enable autonomy and personal responsibility, but it should not be expected prematurely in the treatment process. There is much work to do to unwind neural distortions and physical dependencies before one can start making sound choices for themselves.

Addiction as a Chronic Brain Disease

There is growing consensus among medical professionals that addiction is:

- A function of brain activity and
- Involves changes in brain structure and chemistry.

How addiction plays out in the brain is a complex interplay of chemical reactions and pathway constructions. For the purposes of this discussion, I will focus on the role of dopamine, a 'feel-good' hormone. This process will be explored in greater detail later, but a basic explanation is that pleasurable activities activate the brain's dopamine system. The brain records those activities that bring us pleasure, and release dopamine in order to motivate us to do them again. Over time, if we continue to allow ourselves to be driven by the dopamine hit, the repetition of the activity strengthens the neural pathways associated with it, eventually becoming hard-wired in the brain. Then, the behaviour is performed without conscious thought. It becomes an unchallenged habit.

The problem becomes that man-made stimuli, such as illicit drugs, certain internet activities, and processed foods, deliver dopamine surges that far exceed those produced by natural rewards like eating, social bonding, or sexual activity. Substances like cocaine and methamphetamine directly flood the brain with dopamine, bypassing the gradual and balanced release typical of natural behaviours. For example, drugs like methamphetamine can trigger dopamine levels up to 1,200% higher than the baseline, while natural activities such as eating or sex increase dopamine levels by about 50–200%. Cocaine, for instance, increases dopamine by about 300%, creating a high much stronger than what is experienced through regular rewards like food or social bonding. Similarly, digital interactions such as social media notifications or online gaming exploit neural reward pathways, providing instant gratification that eclipses the slower, more subtle dopamine boosts from connecting with loved ones or achieving personal goals.

The medical definition of a disease is:

"A disorder of structure or function in a human that produces specific symptoms or affects a specific location and is not simply a direct result of physical injury"[9].

In addiction, the brain is the specific location affected, with neurobiological changes causing dependence and reducing the individual's ability to choose. The symptoms of this disease include cravings and withdrawal.

The benefit of seeing addiction as a brain disease is that it helps to reduce the stigma and judgment associated with addiction. It is framed as a condition which can be separated from the character of the person, leading to a more objective perspective:

"I am not addicted; my brain is."

While, as we will see in the following sections, addiction is not that simple, and it spreads much further than just the brain, understanding it as a disease does assist in mitigating the shame that may be preventing progress with treatment. Because when you are in the depths of addiction, any short-term relief from the unbearable sense of shame that comes with it can be helpful.

Additionally, conceptualising addiction as a disease directs the focus towards healing. It shifts the narrative from past mistakes to proactive steps forward, emphasising what can be done to restore brain function. This model also supports the use of medications, which can help manage the neurochemical imbalances caused by addiction, thereby aiding the brain's healing process.

In countries like the United States, where health care is not universally free or subsidised, defining addiction as a chronic brain disease is essential for insurance coverage, enabling access to treatment for millions struggling with addiction. While the disease model is useful for addressing the structural shifts that occur in addiction, it does not address the underlying causes of the initial behaviour, which need to be identified if sustainable healing is to occur.

Moreover, the disease model has been criticised for potentially disempowering individuals by labelling them as helpless patients. Critics argue that it fails to acknowledge the person as a whole—body, mind, and spirit—and may lead to a sense of dependency on medical and psychiatric interventions.

Addiction as a Mental Disorder

The mental disorder model of addiction extends beyond the brain's structural changes to include the thoughts, emotions, and behaviours associated with addiction. According to the World Health Organization (WHO), a disorder is:

"Generally characterised by some combination of abnormal thoughts, emotions, behaviour and relationships with others"[10].

The WHO classifies substance use disorders as mental disorders, with specific criteria outlined in the Diagnostic and Statistical Manual (DSM-5). The DSM presents a comprehensive picture of addiction, considering the physical changes in the brain and the psychological and emotional aspects. The DSM-5 defines substance use disorders as mild, moderate, or severe based on the presence of the following criteria within a 12-month period[11]:

1. Hazardous use: Using the substance in ways that pose a danger to oneself or others.
2. Social or interpersonal problems: Substance use causing conflicts or relationship issues.
3. Neglecting major roles: Failure to meet responsibilities at work, school, or home due to substance use.
4. Withdrawal: Experiencing withdrawal symptoms upon cessation of use.
5. Tolerance: Needing increased amounts of the substance to achieve the same effect.
6. Using larger amounts/longer: Consuming larger quantities or using the substance for extended periods.

7. Repeated attempts to control or quit: Unsuccessful attempts to reduce or stop usage.
8. Much time spent using: Spending excessive time engaging in substance use.
9. Physical or psychological problems: Substance use contributing to health issues.
10. Activities given up: Abandoning activities previously enjoyed in favour of substance use.
11. Craving: Experiencing strong desires or urges to use the substance.

The mental disorder model allows for a more holistic approach to treatment, encompassing both medical and psychological interventions. It acknowledges the complex interplay of brain chemistry, emotional instability, and unhelpful cognitive patterns that can sustain addiction. By addressing these factors, this approach respects the individual as a whole person within their specific context.

However, the mental disorder model also faces challenges, including the stigma associated with mental illness. Although, in reality, the stigma around mental illness is relatively mild compared to that related to addiction. As societal understanding of mental health improves, addiction as a mental disorder is increasingly seen as a component of resilience rather than shame.

Addiction as Deep Learning

Proposed by Professor Marc Lewis, the Deep Learning Model of addiction focuses on the results-oriented aspect of behaviour, suggesting that people learn and repeat actions that effectively achieve their desired outcomes[12]. For instance, someone might initially drink alcohol to relax or cope. In the short-term alcohol achieves these ends, however as a physical dependence develops, this solution becomes the problem.

This model conceptualises addiction as a learned behaviour driven by the need to achieve specific goals, whether they be relaxation, pleasure, or escape. Treatment, therefore, focuses on either:

- Finding healthier goals.
- Developing alternative, healthy behaviours to achieve the same objective.

For example, instead of using alcohol to relax, I could have sought out meditation or yoga classes. The benefits of these behaviours would have well and truly outweighed the instant gratification of the drink, supporting my body, mind and spirit. Note though how much easier and effective it is in the short-term to drink, given its immediate impact and increased hit of dopamine. This is what makes moving away from harmful and addictive behaviours so difficult.

The deep learning perspective straddles the line between the disease and mental disorder models, recognising physical changes in the brain while emphasising behavioural solutions. However, it may not fully address the underlying causes of the emotional and psychological distress that often precede addiction.

A Comprehensive View of Addiction

Each of the models discussed previously contribute valuable insights into the nature of addiction. Rather than viewing them as mutually exclusive, it may be more productive to consider how they interrelate across different stages of the addiction process. As Professor Alison Ritter notes, addiction is a:

"Complex cultural, social, psychological, and biological phenomenon"[13].

No single model captures the entirety of this complexity. Instead, each offers understanding of one part of the addiction picture. In this way, I see that these models, instead of conflicting, complement each other, providing a comprehensive view of the addiction process, as shown in the following diagram.

Figure 1 - How the addiction models fit together

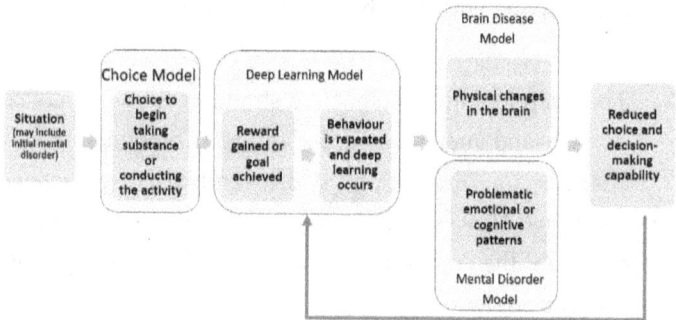

This framework begins with a difficult situation, which may include the struggle with an initial mental disorder. This situation influences the individual's initial choice to engage with a potentially addictive substance or activity, as suggested by the Choice Model. This decision leads to a reward, such as pleasure or relief, reinforcing the behaviour as described in the Deep Learning Model. Over time, the repeated behaviour becomes ingrained, deeply affecting brain function and structure, aligning with the Brain Disease Model.

Additionally, the Mental Disorder Model highlights the role of problematic emotional or cognitive patterns that both contribute to and result from the addictive behaviour. Together, these models illustrate a cyclical and interrelated process where addiction is not solely the result of one factor but a complex interplay of choice, learned behaviours, brain changes, and mental health issues, leading to a reduced capacity for decision-making. This comprehensive view underscores the necessity of multifaceted and holistic treatment approaches that address the biological, psychological and even cultural components of addiction.

Core Concepts

Understanding addiction involves exploring various models, each offering different perspectives that shape treatment approaches.

Addiction as a Choice: This model posits that addiction is a result of personal decisions. However, it often overlooks the diminished decision-making capacity caused by addiction's impact on brain function.

Addiction as a Brain Disease: This viewpoint sees addiction as a chronic condition characterized by changes in brain structure and function, particularly related to the brain's reward system.

Addiction as a Mental Disorder: This model considers addiction within the context of mental health, acknowledging the complex interplay of abnormal thoughts, emotions, behaviours, and social interactions.

Addiction as Deep Learning: This perspective conceptualizes addiction as a learned behaviour that serves a purpose, such as achieving pleasure or relief.

Integrated Approach: Addiction is a multifaceted issue, and each model contributes unique insights into one part of the addiction picture. Together, they provide a more complete understanding of addiction, emphasizing the need for a multi-pronged and multi-layered treatment approach.

Addiction Is a Symptom

As the diagram in the previous chapter shows, all of the models used to explain addiction trace back to a common factor—a difficult situation that the individual attempts to manage through the use of harmful substances or by engaging in unhealthy behaviours.

A symptom is defined as

> *"An indication of the existence of something, especially of an undesirable situation"*[14].

In the context of addiction, this suggests that addiction itself is not the root problem but rather a manifestation of an underlying, undesirable situation. Whether addiction is viewed as a disease, a disorder, or a learned behaviour, it fundamentally represents a response to a deeper issue.

Seeing addiction as a symptom rather than an end in itself invites us to consider the nature of the initial undesirable situation that contributes to addictive behaviours. And so rather than arriving at an answer, we are faced with further, critical questions: What constitutes an undesirable situation? And why do individuals turn to harmful behaviours as a means of coping or escape? These questions point to the need for a more comprehensive understanding of the factors that drive addiction, which will be explored in the next chapter.

Why Do People Become Addicted?

"I have no special talent, I am only passionately curious." ~
Albert Einstein

Understanding why people become addicted is crucial, as it addresses the core of the problem and opens pathways to potential solutions. In previous discussions, addiction was identified as a symptom, a coping mechanism to deal with an undesirable situation. But what exactly is this situation that leads to such extensive psychological and physical challenges? What is the common factor driving individuals towards the self-destructive path of addiction?

Each prevailing model of addiction offers a different perspective:

- The Choice Model tells us that addiction occurs because a person is inherently selfish, weak or morally corrupt.
- The Chronic Brain Disease Model posits that people become addicted because their brain function is compromised.
- The Mental Disorder Model says that people become addicted because they are unable to constructively

deal with distressing emotions and faulty thought patterns.

- The Deep Learning Model argues that people become addicted because they are pursuing unhelpful goals or are taking misguided actions to achieve beneficial goals.

Some people also suggest that addiction could be "in their genes", and so they are physically predisposed to this problem. While certain genetic traits, such as impulsiveness, sensitivity to rejection, and frustration tolerance, may influence addiction, no single gene can be definitively linked to addictive behaviours. This complexity challenges the notion of an "addictive personality," as addiction affects individuals across the personality spectrum—from those who are impulsive and risk-taking to those who are cautious and risk-averse. The only consistent trait among those affected is difficulty in regulating behaviour, and this could be caused by the way a person has been raised, and their early life experiences, not necessarily their genetic makeup.

Given the diverse circumstances of those affected, it might seem impossible, or even stupid to try to pinpoint a singular cause for addiction. However, there are techniques we can employ to find the root cause of a problem, no matter the context in which it occurs. One such technique is 'the five whys', inspired by Warren Berger[15]. The method involves asking 'why' five times in succession to get to the root cause of a problem. Let's apply this technique to the question of why people become addicted:

Why do people become addicted?

Because they keep repeating certain behaviours for example, drinking, taking drugs, gambling or gaming.

Why do they keep repeating the behaviour?

Because it gives them pleasure and distracts them from pain.

Why do they want to distract themselves from pain?

Because they either do not have the ability to deal with it or do not want to deal with it.

Why don't they want to deal with their pain?

Because they feel like they deserve it.

Why would someone feel like they deserve pain?

Because they do not love themselves.

This line of questioning aligns with the perspective of Dr James Hollis[16], who describes addiction as a form of anxiety management. This perspective posits that individuals may not intentionally set out to harm themselves but do so because they lack a sense of their own worth. For example:

- Why would someone consume harmful substances if they truly value their health?
- Why would someone neglect their potential and opportunities if they believed in their abilities?
- Why would someone jeopardise relationships if they felt deserving of love and connection?

The primary question that arises from this insight is: Why do people not love themselves? Marc Lewis[17] identifies a range of potential causes, including stress, shame, trauma, loss, and societal pressures. **My belief is that people do not love themselves because they have been disconnected from their own authentic and life-sustaining spirit.**

There is a radiant source of energy and resilience that we all have, which allows us to make our own unique contribution to this world. This is what I call the spirit. People struggle with self-love because they have lost touch with this source of power and peace. This disconnection can occur when individuals feel pressured to conform to societal standards or achieve external success at the expense of their true selves. Dr Gabor Maté describes this precisely and perfectly as the struggle between attachment and authenticity; we choose clinging to connections rather than allowing our honest selves to shine.

This separation can also occur where people feel they cannot express their authentic selves within their current environment. In that case, a conflict arises between their surroundings and inner spirit. In fact, it puts us at war with ourselves; we begin to hate who we are and we try to suppress our spirit. This conflict causes great pain, which people try to treat through their addiction. As Dr Gabor Maté clearly explains:

"If you look at drugs like heroin, like morphine, like codeine, if you look at cocaine, if you look at alcohol, these are all painkillers. In one way or another, they all soothe

pain. And that's why the real question in addiction is not, 'Why the addiction?,' but, 'Why the pain?'"[18]

This disconnection does not only manifest as addiction but can also lead to other forms of despair, such as anger, materialism, anxiety, depression, and chronic illness. When individuals lose connection with their intrinsic vitality and sense of purpose, it creates a vulnerability to a range of diseases and disorders in the modern world, with addiction being just one outcome.

The Sources of Wellbeing

Dr Richard Davidson and the Centre for Healthy Minds[19] have used neuroscience to research the sources of wellbeing. Their findings, based on extensive studies and experiments, identify four key elements that contribute to holistic health:

1. Awareness: The ability to be mindful and attentive to one's actions.
2. Connection: The capacity for healthy relationships, underpinned by appreciation, kindness, and compassion.
3. Insight: Understanding the beliefs one holds about oneself and how these beliefs shape behaviour.
4. Purpose: A strong sense of meaning and the alignment of daily actions with this purpose.

In addiction, because a person has lost touch with their true spirit, each one of these pillars of wellbeing also becomes compromised:

1. Awareness: As individuals shun their spirits, they lose touch with who they truly are and what they want.
2. Connection: As they see themselves as faulty in some way, they also find it difficult to offer kindness and compassion to themselves, and thus to others.
3. Insight: They twist their beliefs to trap themselves in destructive narratives of powerlessness and unworthiness.
4. Purpose: By moving away from their intrinsic and authentic source of meaning, their sense of purpose also diminishes, making every day actions feel mundane and their life mediocre at best.

In this way it is possible to see how a disconnect with one's spirit starts a cascading effect of causes that negatively impact on a person's whole self and every element of their wellbeing. When one's life feels meaningless and isolated, it creates a significant source of pain which must be treated or numbed in some way. This is where the seeds of addiction are planted.

Ancient Wisdom and Modern Understanding

Many Indigenous cultures and ancient traditions have long recognised the importance of connecting with one's true nature. For instance, the first Australians have a concept known as "gulba-ngi-dyili-nya," which means to know and understand oneself, achieving peace within. This concept is intertwined with "wayamiilbuwawanha," or personal communication, which involves dialogue with one's true self and support from others who nurture the spirit[20].

Similarly, shamanic practices often involve ceremonies for soul retrieval, helping individuals reconnect with the gifts and strengths they were born with but may have lost touch with amid societal pressures[21]. Tibetan traditions also emphasise soul retrieval, which involves rediscovering one's "Buddha Nature"—the inherent kindness and wisdom within each person[22].

Biologist Jeremy Griffith, in his work *Freedom: The End of the Human Condition*[23], suggests that the roots of human suffering may extend back to when humans first gained consciousness. Early humans who questioned the established norms and sought individual paths were often rejected by their communities, leading to feelings of inadequacy and self-doubt. This historical context underscores the broader human struggle with self-acceptance and the consequences of suppressing one's true nature.

The disconnection from one's spirit and the resulting internal conflict manifests in various forms of personal and societal harm, including addiction. When individuals are unable to express their true selves, they attempt to stifle and suppress their spirit, creating a war within themselves. They may resort to self-destructive behaviours as a means of coping with this internal sense of conflict. This self-harm not only impacts their own wellbeing but also denies the wider community the unique contributions and perspectives they have to offer.

Core Concepts

Addiction stems from various factors, including choices, brain changes, mental disorders, and learned behaviours. No single model fully explains why addiction occurs.

Genetics and traits like impulsiveness may play a role, but no specific "addictive personality" or "addiction gene" exists. The common issue is difficulty in behaviour regulation which can be caused by upbringing.

Fundamentally it is a lack of self-love that drives addictive behaviours, as a person does not value themselves enough to avoid harm.

The lack of self-love comes from a disconnect with a person's spirit or true self.

Addiction disrupts key elements of wellbeing—awareness, connection, insight, and purpose—leading to further conflict, dissatisfaction and suffering.

Indigenous and ancient traditions stress the connection with one's true self (spirit) as essential for health and have practices to reunite this essential relationship.

Societal pressures to conform to certain measures of success can lead to self-destructive behaviours, impacting both individual and communal wellbeing.

Why Is There Such a Stigma Around Addiction?

Stigma is defined as:

"a mark of disgrace associated with a particular circumstance, quality, or person."[24]

Despite ongoing efforts to reduce the stigma surrounding addiction—such as initiatives by Rethink Addiction[25] and Addicted Australia[26]—addiction continues to be surrounded by shame and social judgment. This stigma can hinder open discussions about the true causes of addiction and the experiences of those who have struggled with and overcome it. Moreover, the stigma can reinforce a person's view of their lack of self-worth, making them feel like a bad person and making it less likely they will seek help.

We have seen that addiction is not about being a bad person, but is indeed a symptom of deeper distress. So why is it surrounded by such pervasive shame? Why are individuals with addictions often treated as criminals and outcasts? I believe there are four reasons why the stigma around addiction is difficult to decrease:

1. Behavioural Consequences of Addiction

Let's face it, those suffering from addiction do some pretty horrible things. I am the first to admit that while I was in the throes of addiction, my behaviours were disruptive, embarrassing, and burdensome for myself and all those around me. For some, their behaviours during addiction may even cross into violent, dangerous or criminal activities. Because of what they do, individuals with addictions are often ostracised, whether physically, emotionally, or mentally, as others seek to distance themselves from the associated behaviours.

However, there is a difference between what a person does and who they are. While the addiction may characterise them for the moment, it does not define the totality of who they are. Nevertheless, the complexities of addiction are often reduced to simplistic judgments about moral character. This conflation can lead to the belief that individuals with addictions do not deserve the same respect or consideration as those with other illnesses. The addict is judged by their actions, not by the potential that resides underneath.

2. Persistence of the Choice Model

Despite advances in medical research showing that addiction significantly impairs an individual's capacity for choice, the Choice Model persists in public perception. Many still believe that addiction is a self-inflicted condition, viewing those with addictions as responsible for their suffering. This perspective is often reinforced when individuals relapse after receiving help, leading to the assumption that they are unwilling to help themselves or deliberately choosing a path of self-destruction.

This view conveniently simplifies the complex nature of addiction, and how it is driven by a person's context. It also contrasts sharply with how other diseases, such as cancer, are perceived; individuals with cancer are viewed as victims, whereas those with addictions are seen as the perpetrators of their own distress. However, as understanding of the neurological basis of addiction grows, there is hope that this aspect of stigma will diminish, fostering greater empathy for the physiological changes driving addictive behaviours.

3. Association with Mental Illness

Addiction is often classified as a mental illness, which, while beneficial for diagnosis and treatment, does little to alleviate stigma. Although there have been significant efforts to increase understanding and compassion for mental illness, societal discomfort and misconceptions persist. Individuals with mental illnesses are frequently viewed as unstable, irresponsible, or inherently flawed, contributing to a perception that they are weaker or less resilient than those without such conditions.

This stigma not only affects those with mental illnesses but also reinforces feelings of vulnerability and disempowerment among individuals with addictions. It perpetuates the notion that they are fundamentally broken, which can hinder their efforts to reconnect with their sense of strength and agency.

4. Addiction as a Reflection of Vulnerability

Addiction can also evoke discomfort because it exposes vulnerabilities that many people prefer to avoid acknowledging. Encountering individuals who are visibly struggling with addiction—such as those begging for money for a fix, or who are publicly intoxicated—can serve as a stark reminder of our own fears and insecurities. Witnessing such struggles can evoke uncomfortable reflections on one's own life, prompting thoughts about our own weaknesses, failures, lack of control, or unmet needs.

For example, seeing someone struggling with substance use might resonate with personal struggles for meaning or highlight a perceived lack of purpose. There may also be a subconscious envy or frustration—why does this person get to "opt-out" while I have to continue to try and cope with the challenges of everyday life? This reaction can lead to distancing and judgment, as it is easier to label individuals with addictions as "bad" or "weak" than to confront personal discomfort and vulnerability. It is so much more comfortable to tell ourselves that this person is different to us, that is, to deny our common humanity, then to bring forth how much similarity we share.

In these instances, the stigma surrounding addiction functions as a protective mechanism, allowing individuals to maintain a psychological distance from those who are suffering. By categorising people with addictions as fundamentally different or flawed, it becomes easier to navigate daily life without confronting deeper questions about our personal contentment or unresolved pain.

Moving Beyond Stigma

The stigma surrounding addiction is not only damaging to those directly affected but also perpetuates broader misconceptions about human vulnerability and resilience. Each person has the choice to either perpetuate or challenge these stigmas. We all have the ability to perceive those with addictions not as single-dimension sufferers, but as people with great potential. As Sandra Ingerman articulates in *Walking in Light*[27],

---

"You always have the choice to see others as ill or suffering, or in divine light and perfection."

Recognising the shared human experience and the inherent worth of every individual, regardless of their struggles, is a critical step in dismantling the stigma around addiction. Similarly, as we have heard, it is at the heart of healing.

Core Concepts

Stigma is a mark of disgrace associated with a particular circumstance, quality, or person, contributing to shame and social judgment.

Stigma often arises from the embarrassing, disgusting, disruptive, violent and sometimes criminal behaviours linked to addiction.

Despite advances in understanding addiction as a brain disease, many still view it as a choice, perpetuating the belief that individuals are to blame for their condition.

Addiction's classification as a mental illness may not reduce stigma; instead, it often reinforces negative perceptions about instability, irresponsibility, and weakness.

Addiction exposes vulnerabilities that people may find uncomfortable, prompting judgments as a way to distance themselves from their own fears and insecurities.

Reducing stigma requires recognising shared human experiences and valuing individuals beyond their struggles, fostering compassion and understanding in place of judgment.

Section 2-
Understanding the
Healing Pathway

The Addiction Healing Pathway

As previously discussed, it is the disconnection from the spirit, or true self, which is the fundamental cause of addiction. The problem itself sounds simple to correct - reunite with your authentic self. However, the journey to reconnection is not straightforward. Addiction can be likened to a war with many casualties across all areas of an individual's life, and thus, healing requires a comprehensive and sustained approach across the whole human system. The process of addiction, and of it's healing is shown in The Addiction Healing Pathway.

Figure 2 - The Addiction Healing Pathway

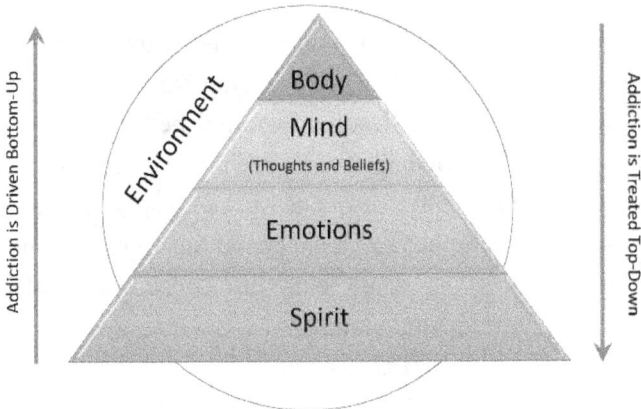

Understanding the Simplicity of the Model

The Addiction Healing Pathway might appear overly simplistic, and this is intentional. It has not been developed to withstand detailed scientific scrutiny. Instead, this model exists to provide individuals, their families, and their support networks with a clear and accessible framework for understanding the healing journey.

It must also not be assumed that because this model is simple, that the healing process it represents is easy. This model serves as map, a guide as to the key steps on the journey. It is not a detailed replica of the terrain across which you will traverse. It is here to provide an overview of the entire landscape, rather than to overwhelm you with intricate detail. It shows you the horizon towards which you are headed, rather than every single hill along the way.

Addiction: A Bottom-Up Process

As shown in The Addiction Healing Pathway, addiction has its roots in the spiritual, developing from a disconnect with one's true self, and leading to diminished self-love and care. The loss of alignment with one's authentic self triggers a cascade of negative emotions, such as fear, shame, and anger, which disrupt the brain's executive functions responsible for decision-making. These emotions create a state of chronic stress, pushing individuals into survival mode—constantly prepared to fight, freeze or flee.

This state of stress and emotional turmoil becomes the undesirable situation that initiates the use of substances or behaviours as a means of temporary relief. It's important to recognise this early stage of addiction, as despite awareness of the potential harm, the compulsion to alleviate suffering can overpower rational judgment, resulting in altered thought patterns that perpetuate the addictive cycle. Over time, these behaviours become ingrained in the brain's circuitry, further entrenching the addiction and leading to additional psychological conditions and physical deterioration.

The disconnection from the spirit and the subsequent emotional and cognitive fallout are not isolated to the individual but extend outward, impacting close relationships and the broader environment. Thus, addiction represents a complex, multi-layered challenge that disrupts not only the person but their entire social and relational context.

Addiction: A Top-Down Healing Approach

While addiction is driven bottom up, healing from addiction occurs top-down, starting with the most immediate and tangible level—the physical body. Healing often begins with detoxification and physical rehabilitation, addressing malnutrition and chemical imbalances that impede cognitive function and emotional regulation. By restoring physical health, individuals gain the energy and clarity needed to engage more deeply in the healing process.

Medications may play a supportive role at this stage, helping to stabilise the body and brain. While there is debate surrounding the pharmaceutical industry's involvement in addiction treatment, appropriate medication, under professional guidance, can be a valuable tool in managing withdrawal symptoms and supporting mental clarity.

Progressing beyond the physical, the next level of focus is the mind—specifically, addressing and reshaping distressing thoughts and beliefs. Cognitive behavioural therapies and other psychological interventions help individuals understand the connections between their thoughts, emotions, and behaviours, fostering the resilience needed to continue their journey.

Emotional healing follows as unresolved feelings of fear, guilt, and anger must be addressed to build the courage necessary for long-term healing. Learning to process and respond to emotions in healthy ways is critical for developing self-compassion and reconnecting with the spirit. The goal is to re-establish a sense of purpose and self-love, culminating in a holistic reconnection with the individual's true self.

Why Present a Pathway?

The Addiction Healing Pathway is presented as a linear progression to provide a clear structure: a defined starting point, a sequential path, and a specific outcome. However, it is acknowledged that in practice, healing is not strictly linear; it involves ongoing interactions and iterations across all levels. Each day may require addressing different aspects of the pathway, as they are all deeply interconnected. The pathway serves as a general guide, with the understanding that true healing is dynamic and individualised.

In the healing process, individuals also often encounter multiple forms of support, with each one working on different parts of the pathway: psychiatrists who focus on faulty thought processes and pharmaceutical treatments, psychologists who address troublesome thoughts and emotions, and other medical specialists who treat physical consequences and conditions. However, without a cohesive framework, it can be challenging to see how these efforts interconnect and contribute to the broader goal of healing. The Addiction Healing Pathway provides a holistic model to guide this process, illuminating the deeply interconnected nature of physical, mental, emotional, and spiritual health in the context of addiction recovery.

Nonetheless, starting with physical health creates a foundation for deeper emotional and spiritual work. It is difficult to fully engage with confronting emotional or spiritual issues without the physical stability and mental clarity provided by the initial stages of healing. The logic of this approach is shown on the following diagram, which highlights how the stages build upon each other.

Figure 3 - The Progression of Healing from Body to Spirit

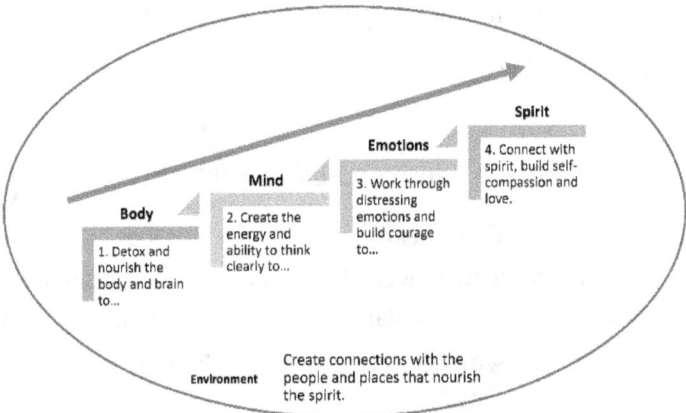

Spirit
4. Connect with spirit, build self-compassion and love.

Emotions
3. Work through distressing emotions and build courage to...

Mind
2. Create the energy and ability to think clearly to...

Body
1. Detox and nourish the body and brain to...

Environment
Create connections with the people and places that nourish the spirit.

The Role of the Environment

The environment, depicted as the surrounding element in the Addiction Healing Pathway, plays a critical role in supporting or hindering healing. This environment includes both the physical and social arenas in which we live. To assist healing, the environment also needs to comprise a comprehensive support system, including:

- Medical and psychiatric professionals to address physical and neurological health.
- Psychologists and counsellors to guide the processing of thoughts and emotions.
- Spiritual mentors or communities to support reconnection with the individual's true nature and sense of purpose.

Simultaneously, it is essential to distance oneself from relationships or environments that enable addictive behaviours. Building a community that reflects and supports one's true self, dreams, and passions can be transformative, providing the encouragement and accountability needed to sustain progress along the pathway.

Addition as a Cause-and-Effect Relationship

The Addiction Healing Pathway provides a clear and empowering framework by illustrating the cause-and-effect nature of addiction, starting from the disconnection from the spirit and cascading through the emotional, mental, and physical realms.

By mapping out the healing pathway in a top-down approach, this model offers a structured way to begin the healing journey. It highlights the importance of addressing immediate physical needs first to build the resilience necessary for deeper emotional and spiritual work.

This step-by-step progression ensures that individuals can systematically rebuild their lives, reconnect with their true selves, and resolve the core issues driving their addiction. By understanding where to begin and how each stage of healing interrelates, this model serves as a practical and holistic guide towards achieving lasting healing and reconnection with one's spirit.

Core Concepts

The Addiction Healing Pathway focuses on the interconnected physical, mental, emotional, and spiritual aspects of healing from addiction.

As shown in The Addiction Healing Pathway, addiction progresses from a disconnection from the true self, leading to emotional turmoil, impaired decision-making, and physical decline, impacting both the individual and their environment.

Healing from addiction begins with a focus on physical health, then addresses mental and emotional wellbeing, ultimately working towards building the energy and courage required to reconnect with the spirit.

Healing is dynamic and non-linear, with the pathway serving as a flexible guide rather than a strict sequence.

A supportive environment, both physical and social, is crucial for sustained healing, emphasising the need for a strong support system.

Blame My Brain!

"Men ought to know that from the brain, and from the brain only, arise our pleasures, joy, laughter and jests, as well as our sorrows, pains, griefs, and tears." ~ Hippocrates

---

The brain plays a significant role in the development and maintenance of addiction. While the brain disease model demonstrates how addiction leads to structural changes in the brain, it is important to recognise that even before addiction takes hold, the way our brains are wired can make us vulnerable to dependency. Fundamentally, humans possess a brain that drives us to seek pleasure and avoid pain. It is this process that can encourage and sustain addictive behaviours.

It's important to note that the discussion of brain structure and function in this chapter is intentionally simplified. The goal is to emphasise understanding of the basic addiction process rather than to transmit technical detail. For those interested in a more comprehensive exploration of addiction's neuroscience, I recommend reading *The Biology of Desire* by Marc Lewis.

The Limbic System and Neocortex

The human brain is a complex organ comprising structures inherited from our reptilian and primate ancestors, overlaid by additional regions that have grown with the evolution of our species. There are two key structures in the brain relevant to our understanding of addiction, and which can be categorised into the:

1. Limbic System
2. Neocortex.

The Limbic System

Located at the core, this includes the brain stem and limbic system, which encompass the hippocampus, amygdala, and hypothalamus. The limbic system houses the brain's pleasure and fear centres. Its primary functions related to addiction involve identifying, remembering, and reacting to pleasurable or threatening experiences. This part of the brain is responsible for instinctual and automatic behaviours that prioritise survival, such as the pursuit of food, safety, and reproduction.

The Neocortex

This includes the outer layers, including the two large cerebral hemispheres or neocortex, responsible for advanced functions such as language, abstract thought, imagination, and consciousness. The neocortex is highly 'neuroplastic ', meaning it can change and adapt over time. This adaptability enables extensive learning and supports complex cognitive processes such as planning, problem-solving, and self-control, which are critical in overcoming addictive impulses but can be overridden by the more primitive drives of the Limbic System.

The challenge lies in the fact that all sensory input first passes through the Limbic System before it reaches the Neocortex, which can predispose individuals to impulsive reactions and addictive behaviours. This structural pathway means that without awareness or intervention, immediate, emotionally driven responses often occur before logical reasoning can intervene.

Figure 4 - The Core Components of the Human Brain

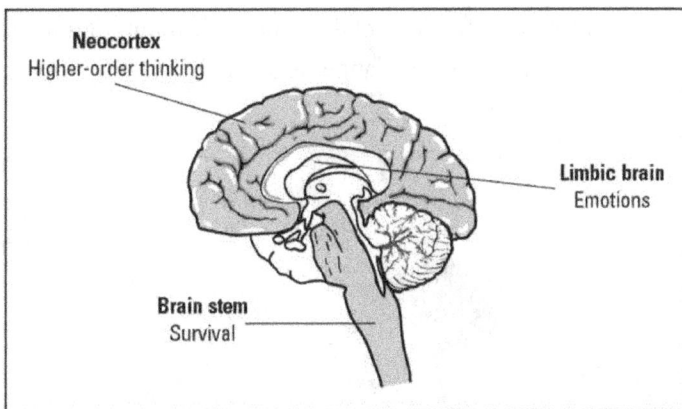

The Limbic System's Influence on Addiction

The Limbic System's primary role is survival, achieved through two basic drives: Seeking pleasure and avoiding pain. These drives underpin much of human behaviour, as Jeremy Bentham summarised:

"Nature has placed humankind under the governance of two sovereign masters, pain and pleasure."

Seeking Pleasure: Facilitated by the neurotransmitter dopamine, this drive motivates behaviours that feel good, such as eating, reproduction, and social bonding. The release of dopamine serves as a reward signal, reinforcing behaviours beneficial for survival and wellbeing.

Avoiding Pain: Through hormones like cortisol and adrenaline, the Limbic System prepares the body to fight, flee, or freeze in response to perceived threats. This drive to avoid pain is fundamental to survival, prompting swift and decisive action when danger is sensed.

Figure 5 - What Our Animal Brain Drives Us To Do

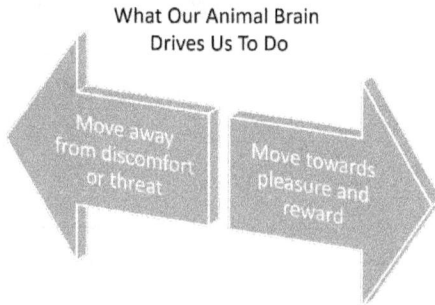

What Our Animal Brain Drives Us To Do

Move away from discomfort or threat

Move towards pleasure and reward

At its core, the Limbic System operates on simplicity: actions that increase pleasure and reduce pain are prioritised. However, in the modern world, where immediate physical threats are less common and artificial sources of pleasure abound, this system can be easily hijacked. The Limbic System's inability to discern between healthy and unhealthy sources of pleasure means that substances and behaviours that offer a high dopamine response—such as drugs, alcohol, and excessive internet use—can become entrenched as primary coping mechanisms, often to the detriment of overall wellbeing.

Prioritising the Greatest Pleasure Hit

The Limbic System prioritises activities that produce the highest dopamine response without distinguishing between healthy and harmful sources. At the same time, natural activities like eating and social interactions trigger dopamine release; substances like drugs and activities like gaming can release far greater amounts, creating stronger motivational drives.

Illicit drugs, for example, can cause up to four times the dopamine release compared to natural rewards, with video games producing dopamine levels comparable to stimulant drugs like amphetamines. As a result, the brain erroneously prioritises these synthetic sources of pleasure, often at the expense of essential activities and relationships. Repeated engagement in these high-dopamine activities 'rewires' the brain's reward system, strengthening the neural pathways associated with addiction. This 'rewiring' leads to the automatic prioritisation of addictive behaviour over more balanced and healthy choices.

This phenomenon explains why individuals may prioritise addictive behaviours over fundamental needs, such as nutrition, sleep, and social connections. The brain's reward system has been rewired to value the immediate and intense pleasure provided by addictive substances or behaviours, often at the expense of long-term health and personal relationships. This misalignment can result in a painful cycle where the individual continues to chase the fleeting rewards of addiction despite the negative consequences on their physical and emotional wellbeing.

When Everything Is a Threat

The flipside of pleasure is pain, and the Limbic System is highly effective at preparing the body and mind to avoid it. However, like its approach to pleasure, the Limbic System does not distinguish between genuine survival threats and perceived threats to one's self-esteem, social status, or emotional wellbeing. It reacts to both with the same intensity, often leading to disproportionate responses to everyday stressors.

Modern life presents numerous situations that the Limbic System can misinterpret as threats, triggering the fight, flight or freeze responses. For example, receiving criticism at work, facing financial difficulties, or experiencing relationship conflicts can all activate the Limbic System's threat response, even though these situations do not immediately threaten one's life. The result is a heightened state of stress and anxiety, which impairs the Neocortex's capacity for rational thought and problem-solving.

When in a state of perceived threat, the body's stress response is activated, releasing cortisol and adrenaline. These hormones prime the body for immediate action but suppress higher cognitive functions, making it difficult to engage in thoughtful decision-making or regulate emotions effectively. In this state, the individual is more likely to seek quick relief from the discomfort, often turning to substances or behaviours that provide an immediate sense of escape or numbing. Over time, this reactive pattern can solidify into an addictive cycle, where the brain increasingly relies on the quick fixes of substances or activities to manage perceived threats.

The Pros and Cons of Neuroplasticity

Neuroplasticity, the brain's ability to reorganise itself by forming new neural connections, is a double-edged sword in the context of addiction. While it enables the brain to adapt and heal, it also allows harmful behaviours to become ingrained. Two key neuroplastic changes in addiction are:

Tolerance: With continued substance use, the brain reduces its dopamine response to protect itself from overstimulation, requiring increasing amounts of the substance to achieve the same effect. This adaptation can escalate addictive behaviours as individuals seek to regain the initial level of pleasure. Tolerance represents the brain's effort to maintain balance in the face of excessive dopamine release, but it inadvertently contributes to the cycle of addiction by driving increased consumption.

Automaticity: Repeated behaviours become automatic, occurring without conscious thought. As with learning to drive or play an instrument, addictive behaviours can become second nature, reducing the individual's ability to make deliberate choices and contributing to the cycle of craving and relapse. This automaticity is reinforced every time the behaviour is repeated in response to a specific cue, such as stress or boredom, creating a strong and lasting association in the brain.

These neuroplastic changes can create significant challenges for healing. As tolerance builds, the individual must consume more of the substance to achieve the desired effect, which can lead to more severe health consequences and deeper psychological dependence. Automaticity further complicates healing by embedding addictive behaviour into daily routines, making it difficult for individuals to break free from established patterns without intentional effort and support.

Implications for Addiction Healing

To counteract the entrenched habits of addiction, the Deep Learning Model suggests redefining goals to focus on achieving pleasure through natural, healthy activities. While this process may take considerable time and effort, it is supported by the brain's neuroplastic potential to develop new, constructive patterns. Activities that promote wellbeing, such as exercise, meditation, and creative pursuits, can stimulate the release of dopamine and other neurotransmitters associated with positive emotions, providing a sustainable source of pleasure that aligns with long-term health.

Furthermore, reconnecting with one's spirit and pursuing a life of meaning and purpose can offer intrinsic rewards that rival the pleasure derived from substances. Living authentically aligns with the Limbic Systems's drive for pleasure but does so through sustainable and fulfilling means, reducing reliance on external sources of gratification. By engaging in activities that resonate with one's values and passions, individuals can cultivate a sense of inner peace and satisfaction that diminishes the appeal of addictive behaviours.

Medication and Brain-Based Treatments

Various medications target the brain's involvement in addiction, offering support in the healing process[28]:

Naltrexone: Reduces the pleasure response to alcohol, making drinking less rewarding. By diminishing the dopamine release associated with alcohol consumption, Naltrexone helps weaken the reinforcement of drinking behaviour, making it easier for individuals to resist cravings.

Disulfiram (Antabuse): Creates an adverse reaction to alcohol, leveraging the brain's fear response to deter use. By inducing severe physical discomfort when alcohol is consumed, Disulfiram taps into the Limbic System's drive to avoid pain, providing a strong deterrent against drinking.

Acamprosate (Campral) and Methadone: Help alleviate cravings by reducing anxiety and promoting relaxation, making it easier to abstain from substance use. These medications work by modulating neurotransmitter systems involved in stress and reward, helping to restore balance in the brain and support healing.

Thiamine (Vitamin B1): Corrects nutritional deficiencies that can exacerbate brain damage from prolonged substance abuse. Thiamine is particularly important in preventing and treating Wernicke-Korsakoff syndrome, a severe neurological disorder associated with chronic alcohol use.

Figure 6 - MRI of a Healthy Brain vs Brain with WKS

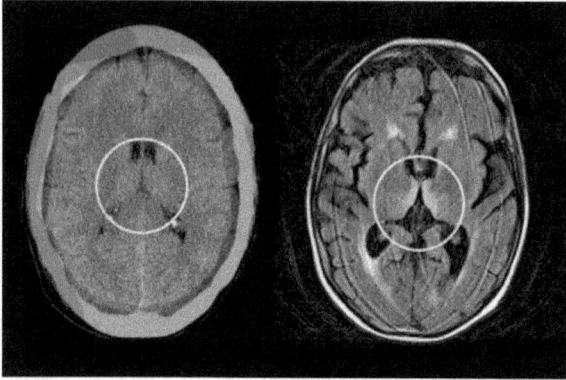

Wernicke-Korsakoff Syndrome (WKS)

While medications can aid healing, they cannot reverse all damage, particularly if addiction persists unchecked. Conditions like Wernicke-Korsakoff syndrome highlight the importance of early intervention to prevent irreversible brain damage.

Wernicke-Korsakoff Syndrome (WKS) is composed of two distinct but related conditions: Wernicke's encephalopathy and Korsakoff's psychosis.

- Wernicke's encephalopathy is characterised by symptoms such as confusion, ataxia (loss of coordination), and ophthalmoplegia (eye movement abnormalities).
- If left untreated, Wernicke's encephalopathy can progress to Korsakoff's psychosis, which primarily affects memory, leading to severe short-term memory loss, confabulation (fabricating memories), and difficulty learning new information.

Early recognition and treatment with thiamine supplementation are crucial, as WKS can cause permanent brain damage and is potentially life-threatening if not addressed promptly.

Core Concepts

The brain's inherent drives for pleasure and pain avoidance creative a vulnerability towards addiction.

Addiction develops when the brain's pleasure responses are hijacked by substances or behaviours that release high levels of dopamine.

The brain misreads these high dopamine substances or behaviours as essential for survival and so prioritises them above natural and healthy pursuits.

Neuroplasticity enables the brain to adapt and change, which can lead to both the reinforcement of addictive behaviours (automaticity) and the potential for healing through building new, healthier habits.

Addiction's entrenchment in the brain involves processes like tolerance (requiring more of a substance for the same effect) and automaticity (ingrained behaviours), which complicate the healing journey.

Healing from addiction involves retraining the brain to seek pleasure in natural, fulfilling activities and reconnecting with one's true self to find intrinsic, sustainable rewards.

The Immediate Healing Concerns

"To change your life, you need to change your priorities." ~ Mark Twain

The pivotal role our bodies play is often overlooked, with many people viewing our physical form merely as merely a tool to achieve desired outcomes. Attention to the body typically arises only when there is a crisis, when it begins to falter or hinder personal ambitions. However, the body is a remarkable and complex system that, when respected and properly cared for, can provide strength, energy, and wisdom. It serves as a crucial vehicle for connecting with one's true and unique spirit.

The body contributes to overall wellbeing in several key ways, such as:

- Providing fuel for the brain, which enables clear thinking and sound decision-making.
- Supplying energy needed to pursue passions and engage in daily activities.
- Facilitating rest and restoration, which are essential for the healing journey.
- Allowing for self-expression through movement and physical actions.
- Creating connections with the physical world and other people through sensory experiences.
- Enabling the experience of sensations and enhancing emotional and spiritual understanding.

However, addiction inflicts significant damage on the body, both physically and mentally. This damage can be both acute and chronic, resulting from prolonged exposure to toxic substances or maladaptive behaviours. The path to healing, therefore, begins with immediate and focused care for the body in order to provide a solid foundation for addressing the emotional and spiritual levels of the pathway.

The First Step – Withdrawal

Withdrawal marks the first critical step in physical healing. Due to the nature of addiction, both the body and brain develop dependencies on substances, or the highs derived from addictive behaviours. As discussed in the previous chapter, the brain re-prioritises these substances or activities over all other human needs. Thus, withdrawal can be seen as stripping away the addiction's lifeline, prompting the body and brain to resist fiercely.

Withdrawal symptoms vary widely in intensity and duration. The acute phase lasts a few weeks, while milder, chronic symptoms may persist for months. Common symptoms of withdrawal include[29]:

- Cravings for the addictive substance or activity
- Anxiety and restlessness
- Fatigue and mood swings
- Nightmares and sleep disturbances
- Headaches and sweating
- Loss of appetite and gastrointestinal distress.

While these symptoms are often moderate, they can be profoundly uncomfortable and pose a challenge to commitment during detoxification. The body's response to the absence of the addictive substance often drives an intense desire to relieve the discomfort, reinforcing the cycle of substance use.

For some individuals, withdrawal can trigger more severe and potentially life-threatening symptoms, such as:

- Severe depression or anxiety
- Paranoia and psychosis
- Suicidal ideation or self-harm
- Rapid heart rate and high body temperatures
- Delirium tremens (severe alcohol withdrawal)
- Seizures and convulsions.

Given the potential severity of these symptoms, it is crucial to have some level of medical support during withdrawal. Levels of medical involvement can vary based on individual needs and risks, ranging from outpatient supervision to fully managed inpatient care with medication support. The main options when it comes to withdrawal support are as follows:

- Medical Supervision: Regular outpatient visits or check-ups with a general practitioner.
- Medical Monitoring: Inpatient care where medical staff regularly check the patient's progress.
- Medically Managed: Inpatient care with the use of medications to manage withdrawal symptoms and support the detox process.

Figure 7 - The Levels of Medical Support During Withdrawal

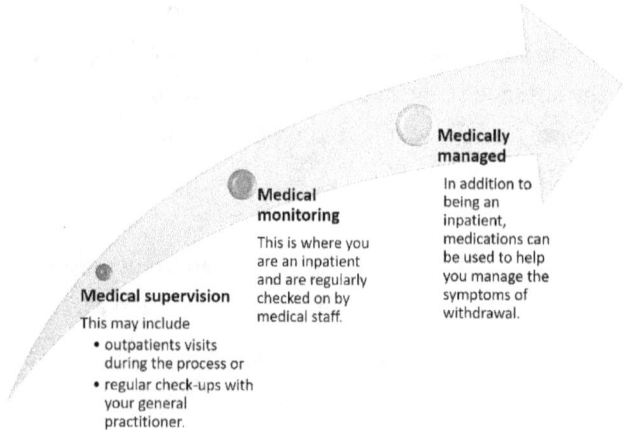

Medically managed

In addition to being an inpatient, medications can be used to help you manage the symptoms of withdrawal.

Medical monitoring

This is where you are an inpatient and are regularly checked on by medical staff.

Medical supervision

This may include

- outpatients visits during the process or
- regular check-ups with your general practitioner.

Addressing the Physical Damage

Addiction can leave a lasting imprint on the body and brain, with some effects being temporary while others may be permanent. Prolonged substance abuse can lead to severe physical consequences, including ongoing psychosis associated with certain drug use. The toxic environment created within the body by addiction can also foster a range of cancers, such as liver, throat, lung, stomach, breast, and renal cancers. Conditions like ulcers, pancreatitis, heart disease, neuropathic disorders, hepatitis, and psoriasis are common among individuals struggling with addiction, particularly when liver function is compromised.

Additionally, chronic addiction often results in significant nutritional deficiencies. A body deprived of proper nutrition is less capable of repairing itself, leading to further complications and an overall decline in health.

Establishing a strong medical support team is critical in addressing these issues. The first important task is to find a knowledgeable and compassionate general practitioner. They can develop a treatment plan and help coordinate care with specialists, such as nutritionists, hepatologists, cardiologists, and mental health professionals. This plan should focus on identifying the extent of physical and mental damage and outlining steps to address these challenges through targeted interventions.

While the extent of damage caused by addiction can be daunting, it is important to remember that this health assessment is not the endpoint—it is merely the beginning. Understanding and accepting the current state of health is a critical step in healing, allowing for action and the necessary changes to improve wellbeing. Even if some damage cannot be completely healed, pursuing self-compassion and care can significantly improve the quality of life.

Navigating the Emotional and Mental Toll

One of the greatest challenges individuals face when addressing the physical damage of addiction is the emotional toll that accompanies a health assessment. Realising the extent of harm done can lead to feelings of guilt, shame, and despair, particularly if some conditions are irreversible. It is common for individuals to grapple with self-blame and anger over the choices that led to their current state, and this emotional burden can be overwhelming.

However, it is vital to reframe this narrative. The focus should not be on what has been lost or damaged but on the opportunity that lies ahead. Every effort made toward healing and self-care is a step away from self-destruction and toward a future defined by resilience and growth. Embracing this mindset can foster a renewed commitment to healing, enabling full engagement with treatment plans and support systems.

Practical Steps for Physical Healing

Healing from addiction requires a holistic approach that addresses not only the immediate withdrawal symptoms but also the long-term health effects. Key steps include:

Nutritional Support: A balanced diet rich in vitamins and minerals can help repair the damage caused by addiction. Working with a nutritionist can provide personalised guidance on rebuilding nutritional stores, addressing deficiencies, and optimising overall health.

Hydration: Proper hydration is essential for flushing out toxins and supporting bodily functions. Alcohol and drug use can severely dehydrate the body, so prioritising water intake is crucial especially during detox.

Movement: Regular physical activity can enhance mood, increase energy levels, and support overall physical health. Exercise stimulates the release of endorphins and other neurotransmitters that can improve mental wellbeing and help combat the fatigue often experienced during healing.

Rest and Sleep: Quality sleep is vital for the body's repair processes and for managing stress levels. Establishing a consistent sleep routine can aid in restoring normal sleep patterns, which are often disrupted by addiction.

Medical Monitoring: Regular check-ups and ongoing monitoring by healthcare professionals can help track progress and address emerging health concerns. Early intervention is key to managing potential complications and ensuring a smooth healing process.

The Path Forward

Acknowledging the physical damage caused by addiction is a difficult experience, but it also offers empowerment. It allows for the creation of a targeted plan to rebuild and restore the body to its optimal state. This process is not just about healing the damage but also about fostering a new relationship with the body—one rooted in respect, care, and understanding.

As the journey continues, it is never too late to choose self-compassion. The road to healing is paved with small, intentional steps toward better health and wellbeing. Each positive choice contributes to rewiring the brain and bringing forth a person's full potential.

It is better late than never.

Core Concepts

Addiction causes significant damage to the body, mind and spirit, all of which must be addressed for effective healing.

Withdrawal is the first step in physical healing, and it involves the body adjusting to the absence of addictive substances or behaviours, with symptoms ranging from mild to severe.

Medical support during withdrawal is crucial, with options ranging from outpatient supervision to fully managed inpatient care.

Addiction may lead to other various health issues, including cancers, heart disease, and nutritional deficiencies, requiring a strong medical support team for comprehensive care.

Addressing the physical damage involves recognising the current state of health as the starting point for targeted interventions and self-care.

Healing also requires addressing the emotional toll of health assessments, reframing the focus from guilt to opportunity for growth and resilience.

Practical steps for physical healing include nutritional support, hydration, physical activity, rest, and regular medical monitoring.

Embracing a holistic approach to healing fosters a renewed relationship with the body, rooted in care and respect, and supports the path towards overall wellbeing.

Section 3- Healing Body and Mind

Setting Up Base Camp

"Build a strong base. The journey to peaks of excellence requires a strong base camp." ~ C.N. Rao

Healing from addiction can be compared to the process of learning to live anew. During the period of addiction, and often well before its onset, individuals often become adept at isolation and self-avoidance. Consequently, like a child learning to walk or read, the healing journey begins with the basics. As The Addiction Healing Pathway outlines, this process starts with the most fundamental aspect—the body. When individuals treat their bodies well—nourishing and respecting them—they can create a foundation for the growth of energy and wisdom.

Before embarking on a difficult climb, mountaineers establish what is known as a Base Camp. Base Camp serves several purposes, including providing a secure location to prepare for the climb, storing supplies that can be readily accessed during the expedition, and offering a refuge during times of danger. By viewing the healing process as an expedition, it becomes clear that establishing healthy habits that support the body and mind form the Base Camp for the healing journey.

Based on practical experience, there are five essential elements that contribute to creating a solid foundation for this journey. These elements require deliberate development and a lifelong commitment to sustaining them. They include:

1. Breath
2. Nutrition
3. Sleep
4. Movement
5. Medication (if necessary).

Figure 8 - Setting Up Base Camp

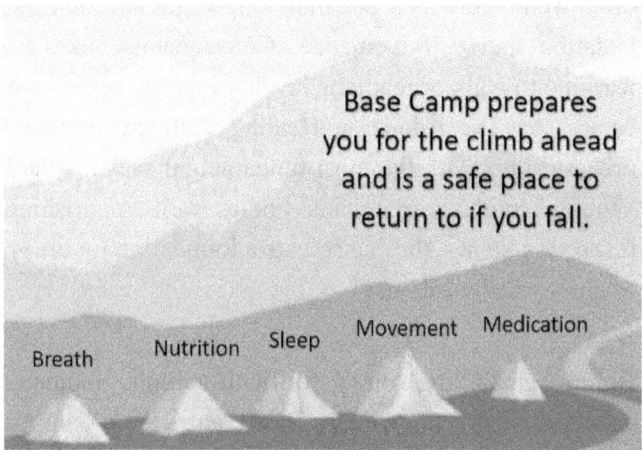

Base Camp prepares you for the climb ahead and is a safe place to return to if you fall.

Breath   Nutrition   Sleep   Movement   Medication

Without these five essentials in place, the journey out of addiction can become significantly more challenging and exhausting. It is, therefore, advisable to remain at Base Camp as long as necessary to build the strength and clarity required to move forward.

Climbers do not seek to hastily ascend a vast mountain. They stay at base camp until their bodies have acclimatised to the altitude and they have organised themselves sufficiently for the adventure ahead. Similarly, embarking on the significant journey of The Addiction Healing Pathway without securing a strong foundation can be detrimental to the traveller's safety and success. Although the consequences may not be as severe as those faced by unprepared mountaineers on Mount Everest, having a robust foundation of basic practices can influence the healing process and its outcomes.

However, Base Camp should not be viewed solely as an initial step; it also serves as a reliable place to return whenever there is a need to regroup and refocus. If a setback occurs, a well-established Base Camp can prevent further regression. It contains all the necessary components to regain strength and resume the ascent without having to start over. For example, in the event of a lapse, if sound habits are in place concerning breathing, eating, sleeping, exercise, and medication, healing can be relatively swift and less distressing. However, without these foundational practices, individuals may become disoriented, confused, and vulnerable, increasing the risk of further setbacks or continued regression. Without Base Camp, a person may find themselves slipping down the hill even further.

Breath

Despite being a fundamental force, the power of the breath is often taken for granted until it is compromised, such as during a panic attack or a severe asthma episode. Beyond the essential function of sustaining life, breath can serve as a tool for self-regulation, offering ways to calm in moments of distress, clear the mind for decision-making, ground the body in the present moment, and energise the individual to move forward.

Breathing also plays a vital role in cellular respiration, a process by which cells convert oxygen and nutrients into usable energy. If breathing is inadequate, the resulting oxygen deficiency can impair cellular energy production, leading to mental and physical fatigue. This exhaustion can hinder clarity and impede decision-making, both essential in the healing journey. Furthermore, deep breathing exercises can activate the parasympathetic nervous system, the body's relaxation response, which is beneficial when encountering distressing emotions commonly experienced during healing.

Nutrition

Nutritional support is a critical component of healing. There are two primary principles to consider in setting up your nutritional base camp:

1. When to eat and
2. What to eat.

Regular mealtimes can help maintain stable blood glucose levels, which is essential in preventing vulnerabilities contributing to relapse. Consistent mealtimes ensure that the brain receives a steady supply of energy necessary for making constructive decisions throughout the day. Scheduling meals approximately five hours apart can help prevent the adverse effects of low blood sugar, including brain fog, irritability, and headaches, all of which can undermine the capacity for sound decision-making that is vital to healing. When one is not thinking clearly it is a real risk that they will revert to harmful habits rather than make conscious choices to undertake helpful behaviours.

Individuals' dietary choices should align with their unique physical and mental health needs at any given time. There is no absolute prescription for right or wrong foods, as requirements vary depending on circumstances. For instance, if an individual is recovering from a physically demanding situation, quick energy sources like electrolyte drinks may be preferable. Conversely, after a less demanding day, a balanced meal rich in protein and vegetables would be more appropriate for nourishment before an overnight fast.

Food also plays a significant emotional role, influencing feelings and behaviours. Recognising these associations can guide more intentional dietary choices that support both physical and emotional wellbeing. It is recommended that individuals consider including a naturopath or dietitian in their support team to help develop a personalised eating plan. These professionals can provide guidance but also accountability to ensure that a person is sticking to the meal plans that give them the best chance of success.

Sleep

Sleep is universally acknowledged as crucial for both physical and mental restoration, making it an essential aspect of repairing the damage associated with addiction. Quality sleep facilitates the brain's natural detoxification processes, allowing cerebrospinal fluid to clear away waste products that accumulate during wakefulness[30]. In this way, sleep is like the deep clean function for our brain, and adequate sleep therefore is critical for cognitive function, emotional regulation, and overall physical vitality—all of which are necessary for sustained healing.

Maintaining good sleep hygiene—such as adhering to consistent sleep and wake times, minimising screen exposure before bed, and establishing a calming bedtime routine—supports the body's need for restorative rest. Poor sleep can have significant negative impacts, including increased emotional reactivity and reduced capacity to handle the daily challenges of healing. Therefore, prioritising sleep is a critical investment in the healing journey.

Movement

Rather than use the concept of exercise, the notion of movement is far more helpful. Exercise comes with the associations of specific repetitive activities, and the experience of boredom and deflating discipline. Whereas movement can be found in so many enjoyable activities. It is movement, not just "exercise" that contributes to physical, mental and spiritual health. Engaging in continuous moderate-intensity movement for about 20 minutes, such as walking, dancing, or yoga, can trigger the release of mood-enhancing chemicals like endorphins and endocannabinoids. Regular movement is associated with increased happiness, a greater sense of purpose, and enhanced social connectivity, which can help counter the isolation and loneliness that are common in addiction[31].

Movement also supports multiple aspects of The Addiction Healing Pathway. Physically, it aids in experiencing and expressing joy, offering a natural countermeasure to anhedonia—a condition often experienced during early healing. Mentally, the persistence required in physical activity can challenge entrenched beliefs and behaviours associated with addiction, fostering confidence in a person's ability to stick to a course of action and to persist despite obstacles. Spiritually, movement can promote self-expression and enhance social connections, assisting individuals in finding their place in the world and reaching their full potential.

Medication

The role of medication in healing is complex and varies based on individual needs. Medication can be an important tool when used with clear objectives, such as stabilising mood, managing cravings, or addressing specific health conditions. It is crucial for individuals to engage in transparent discussions with healthcare providers to understand the purpose and expected outcomes of any prescribed medications. Medication should be seen as just one component of a comprehensive healing plan rather than as a "magic pill" or singular solution.

The effectiveness of medication should be regularly evaluated, and adjustments should be made as necessary to ensure that it continues to support the broader healing process. Commitment to following prescribed regimens and monitoring progress with healthcare professionals is vital for achieving the intended therapeutic outcomes.

Beginning At Base Camp

Establishing a Base Camp involves creating a solid foundation of self-care practices that support physical and mental health, providing a stable platform from which to launch and sustain the healing journey. By seeking to improve and integrating breath, nutrition, sleep, movement, and medication, individuals can develop the strength and clarity needed to navigate the complexities of healing from addiction. Base Camp serves not only as a starting point but also as a reliable refuge that can be revisited in times of challenge, providing the necessary means to regain stability and continue progressing toward long-term healing.

Core Concepts

Base Camp serves as a foundation for the healing journey, providing stability and essential resources, similar to how mountaineers prepare for a challenging climb.

Establishing a solid Base Camp involves developing five key self-care elements: breath, nutrition, sleep, movement, and medication.

Breath is fundamental for self-regulation, energy, calmness and clarity in decision-making.

Nutrition supports stable blood sugar levels, critical for mental clarity and resilience.

Sleep facilitates brain detoxification and restoration, crucial for cognitive function, emotional regulation, and physical health.

Movement provides physical and mental benefits, releasing mood-enhancing chemicals and countering feelings of isolation; it fosters resilience and self-expression.

Medication, when needed, should be used purposefully and in consultation with healthcare providers to support specific goals.

A well-established Base Camp not only supports initial progress but also offers a reliable place to return to during setbacks, ensuring ongoing strength throughout the healing journey.

We Become our Beliefs

"Beliefs have the power to create and the power to destroy."
~ Tony Robbins

In the progression of The Addiction Healing Pathway, there is a shift from addressing the tangible and physical effects of addiction to exploring the subtle and mental factors that perpetuate self-destructive behaviours. While modifying behaviours is crucial, without an understanding of the beliefs that are beneath them, we are flying blind. We can attempt to make change, but are only guessing at whether it will work. Moreover, unidentified or unchallenged beliefs can sabotage the healing process and we would be no wiser as to what had gone wrong. Just as diagnostic tests such as scans and blood tests can be uncomfortable but necessary, examining one's beliefs is an essential step that can help us make effective shifts in our lives.

What Are Beliefs?

A belief is defined as a thought, attitude, or opinion that an individual accepts as true. Many of our beliefs are adopted from our parents and carers, ingrained in childhood. However, some are also formed through our own life experiences, with our time away from our families potentially being used to discredit or dispose of those we were taught when we were young.

It is important to note that a belief does not have to be based in fact. All that matters for a belief to be influential over a person's behaviour is the individual's acceptance of it as truth. The impact of beliefs is well-illustrated by placebo research, where even if a person is given a simple sugar pill, it can trigger real physiological responses. It only requires a person to believe that they have been given an effective treatment to result in improvements in conditions such as pain, fatigue, coughs, erectile dysfunction, and even Parkinson's disease. When an individual truly believes in the efficacy of a treatment, it becomes their reality and results in tangible outcomes.

The Power of Beliefs

Beliefs that are accepted as truth significantly influence all aspects of our lives, including thoughts, emotions, and behaviours. This impact is shown by the Cognitive Behavioural Therapy Model.

Figure 9 - The Cognitive Behavioural Therapy Model

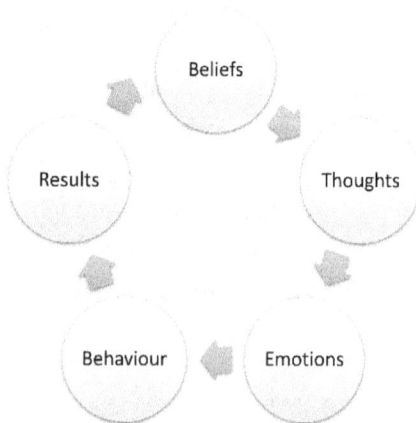

Let's work through the impact of beliefs through an example. Consider the case of a person offered a place in a rehabilitation program. This is one possible pathway.

Belief: I am a hopeless case.

Thought: If I try this, I am likely to fail.

Emotion: Despair and fear.

Behaviour: Minimal engagement in the program, maintaining a guarded and closed attitude towards staff.

Result: Limited benefit from the program, reinforcing the belief that the effort was futile and discouraging future attempts at rehabilitation.

In this scenario, the belief acts as a self-fulfilling prophecy, reinforcing a cycle of negative outcomes. In contrast, consider what may happen if the person enters into the same scenario with a different belief.

Belief: I am not hopeless; I just need to find the right help.

Thought: This rehab may provide the help I need.

Emotion: Optimism and curiosity.

Behaviour: Active engagement in the program, asking questions, and forming relationships with staff.

Result: A positive experience, even if modest, leads to an openness to future help.

These examples illustrate how different beliefs can lead to dramatically different outcomes, emphasising the importance of examining and potentially reshaping beliefs to support healing efforts.

"The outer conditions of a person's life will always be found to reflect their inner beliefs." ~ James Allen

The Most Harmful Beliefs

Beliefs regarding external factors such as education, finances, relationships, diet, and career significantly influence one's actions and life outcomes. However, the beliefs one holds about the self can either make or break one's ability to heal from addiction.

"You are what you believe yourself to be." ~ Paulo Coelho

I Am Unworthy

The most harmful belief a person can have as they are trying to heal from addiction is that they are unworthy of health and of happiness. As we have seen, this belief is not only behind the initial foray into self-destructive behaviours, but it can inhibit the changes necessary to heal. This belief, while integral in addiction can also manifest in many other ways, such as enduring unhealthy relationships, neglecting mental health, or persisting in unfulfilling careers.

When individuals perceive themselves as unworthy, it can trigger a downward spiral of self-neglect and harm. This belief may drive a person to self-medicate through substances or addictive behaviours to fill an internal void. As addiction takes hold, the belief in unworthiness can inhibit the pursuit of healing resources, reinforce isolation from support systems, and perpetuate harmful relationships. This belief can even lead to self-sabotage when progress is made, undermining achievements to maintain a perceived status of inadequacy.

My Worth Depends On Others

Another related and harmful belief is that one's worth is contingent upon external validation from others. This belief can present as a reliance on a partner for a sense of self-worth or a compulsive need for approval and recognition from figures such as parents, peers, or employers. In these instances, self-worth is externally defined, leading to a precarious sense of identity that is vulnerable to external criticism or rejection. For if validation from another is withdrawn, the person's sense of self is shattered, and they may fall into a belief that they are inherently flawed.

The Painful Realisation

Ask yourself this question right now - "Do I believe I am worthy of health and happiness?"

If the answer is no, then I suspect this realisation may be deeply painful. Seeing the belief that we see ourselves as unworthy is often described as one of the most profound emotional wounds, for with this comes the understanding that we are the cause of our own suffering. Acknowledging oneself as both the victim and the perpetrator of self-sabotage can be a source of intense distress.

Despite the discomfort that comes with this recognition, it is also a pivotal moment of empowerment. Understanding the detrimental beliefs that have governed past behaviours opens the opportunity to consciously redefine one's beliefs and, in turn, alter the trajectory of one's healing journey. By challenging and reshaping beliefs about worthiness and capability, individuals can reclaim agency and foster a more constructive and hopeful path forward. This can be done through self-reflection, therapy, or support groups, where individuals can share their beliefs and experiences and receive feedback and guidance on how to challenge and reshape their beliefs. The next chapter will provide some practical techniques that you can use to test your beliefs as they arise.

Core Concepts

Beliefs are thoughts or attitudes accepted as true, influencing actions, emotions, and outcomes, regardless of their factual accuracy.

In addiction healing, underlying beliefs can significantly impact the process, with negative beliefs often reinforcing self-destructive behaviours and hindering progress.

Common harmful beliefs in addiction include feelings of unworthiness or lack of control, often leading to self-neglect and perpetuating addiction.

Acknowledging and challenging detrimental beliefs about oneself is crucial for empowerment and healing, allowing individuals to redefine their self-perception and reclaim control over their healing journey.

Reshaping beliefs can be facilitated through self-reflection, therapy, and supportive environments that encourage the exploration and reformation of personal beliefs.

Understanding the power of beliefs and actively working to align them with healing goals can transform the healing process, leading to more positive and sustainable outcomes.

You Are Not Your Thoughts

"All that we are is a result of what we have thought." ~ Buddha

The healing journey from addiction is a deeply personal and unique process, varying from person to person. However, one aspect of the journey can be anticipated with certainty: the presence of troubling thoughts. It's important to remember that these thoughts are a normal part of the human experience, rooted in the evolutionary function of the brain, which is constantly seeking to help us preserve energy, scanning for threats and preparing us to take action. Our brains are wired to protect us, and this can manifest in thoughts such as:

"It is too hard."
"I give up."
"I can't cope."
"I deserve this."

These thoughts are normal, reflecting the brain's efforts to navigate the dangers that it perceives, even if they are not real. However, there is one crucial thing that you must understand.

"You are not your thoughts." ~ Eckhart Tolle

Recognising that you are not your thoughts can be transformative and can facilitate a significant shift in your relationship with your inner dialogue.

Understanding Your Thoughts

Thoughts are the product of interactions between electrical impulses and chemicals in the brain. When one neuron transmits a signal to another, this communication can manifest as a thought. Recent research suggests that the average adult experiences approximately 6,000 thoughts each day, translating to around 400 thoughts per waking hour or over six thoughts per minute. Given the sheer volume of thoughts, it is unsurprising that individuals may feel overwhelmed at times.

Many of these thoughts occur subconsciously and pertain to basic physiological needs such as hunger, thirst, body regulation, and potential threats. It is estimated that about 95% of thoughts are subconscious, leaving approximately 5% that reach conscious awareness. Practically speaking, this means that a conscious thought emerges every few minutes, requiring some degree of cognitive processing. While increasing awareness of thoughts is beneficial, it is equally important to develop strategies for dealing with thoughts already within our conscious awareness.

Responding to Thoughts

Thoughts, in and of themselves, do not possess intrinsic power. Similar to beliefs, they only gain influence when we engage with them, allowing them to shape our feelings and behaviours. Therefore, when faced with troubling thoughts, we are also presented with a choice:

1. Engage with the thoughts and potentially spiral into a cognitive loop
2. Neutralise the thoughts through conscious and compassionate responses.

Engaging in Cognitive Loops

A cognitive loop occurs when an individual becomes entangled in a negative thought pattern, allowing it to escalate into distressing emotions and unhelpful actions and potentially leading to a cycle of relapse. For example:

Thought: "I am hopeless. I can't cope. I need something to ease the pain."

Feeling: Fear, desperation, and desire.

Action: Engaging in the substance or behaviour.

Result: A relapse and sense of failure.

Belief: Reinforced perception of hopelessness.

Thought: "I can't do this. I can't cope without my substance or activity."

Feeling: Guilt, shame, despair.

Action: Re-engaging in the substance or behaviour to alleviate these feelings.

This cycle can perpetuate for extended periods, often years, resulting in profound personal and relational consequences. Let's examine how to neutralise such thoughts to prevent them from dictating our behaviours.

Neutralising Difficult Thoughts

Neutralising difficult thoughts involves a three-step process: noticing, naming, and neutralising[32].

Step 1: Notice

The first step is to become aware of the thoughts as they occur. Mindfulness allows recognising when a thought arises and pausing before reacting. This process may seem straightforward, but it demands practice, especially during moments of vulnerability, such as when an individual is tired or emotionally distressed. During these times, when we have less energy for awareness, it becomes easier for them to take hold. So, whenever we are able to stop and see a thought occurring, it is a cause for celebration. Because it is a significant step forward to countering those thoughts that will hold us back from healing.

Step 2: Name

By naming a thought, you create a separation between the thought and who you truly are. A simple yet powerful phrase to use is:

"I am having the thought that..."

This practice helps to maintain perspective and prevent thoughts from becoming entangled with your self-concept. By acknowledging the thought as a transient mental event, you can assess it more objectively.

Step 3: Neutralise

Once a thought has been noticed and named, it can be further neutralised through one of three methods, each requiring different levels of cognitive engagement:

- **Questioning the helpfulness**: Ask whether the thought is beneficial to your healing journey. If the answer is no, dismiss the thought without further engagement. This approach allows you to make a conscious choice not to let the thought influence your actions.

- **Disputing the validity**: Some thoughts are persistent and may require further scrutiny. In such cases, challenging the thought's accuracy can be effective. For instance, if the thought is "I am a bad person," counter it by recalling instances of kindness, generosity, and positive actions you have taken. Recognise that human behaviour is multifaceted, and no single thought can encapsulate the entirety of one's character.

- **Deciding on action**: For thoughts that persist despite attempts to dismiss or dispute them, using a Decision-Making Matrix can help determine the appropriate response. This model considers the importance of the issue and the level of control you have over it, guiding you in deciding whether to take action or let go.

The Decision-Making Matrix

The Decision-Making Matrix (shown in the diagram below) is useful for navigating persistent thoughts by assessing their significance and controllability. For example, suppose you are worried that others are judging you unfavourably because they know you have struggled with addiction. In that case, the matrix can help clarify that:

- Others' opinions of you are important at this time, however
- You have no ability to control what other people think of you, therefore
- The most helpful course of action is to focus on staying true to your values.

Living in accordance with your values will provide a sense of fulfilment and allow you to keep a more helpful perspective on external judgments.

Figure 10 - The Decision-Making Matrix

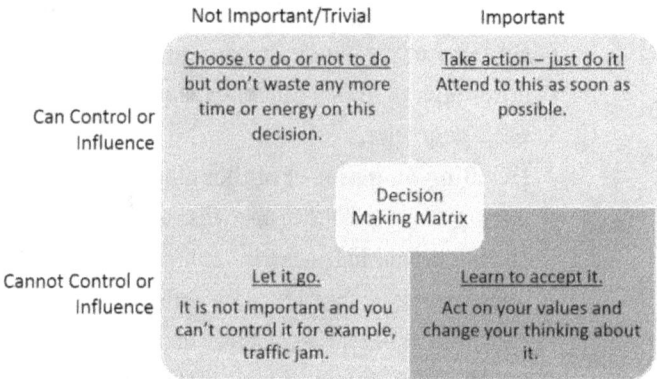

	Not Important/Trivial	Important
Can Control or Influence	Choose to do or not to do but don't waste any more time or energy on this decision.	Take action – just do it! Attend to this as soon as possible.
Cannot Control or Influence	Let it go. It is not important and you can't control it for example, traffic jam.	Learn to accept it. Act on your values and change your thinking about it.

Decision Making Matrix

"If there is something you can do about it...why worry? If there is nothing you can do about it...why worry?" ~ *Buddhist proverb*

Identifying Harmful Thought Patterns

Certain thought patterns can be particularly detrimental to progress on the healing path. Common phrases that often signal unhelpful thoughts include:

- I should...
- I should not...
- I must...
- I must not...
- I have to...
- I always...
- I never...
- I can't...

These expressions create rigid, black-and-white perceptions that can obstruct creativity and problem-solving. They reinforce feelings of guilt, shame, and powerlessness, which are counterproductive to healing. For example, after a relapse, a thought such as "I always fail" can entrench a sense of inevitability and prevent individuals from exploring alternative, more constructive responses.

Transforming Limiting Thoughts

Transforming limiting thoughts into empowering ones involves replacing restrictive language with terms emphasising choice and agency. Consider substituting phrases like:

- I will...
- I decide...
- I choose...
- I want to...

- I choose not to...

These alternatives foster a sense of control and possibility, shifting the narrative from victimhood to empowerment. For instance, instead of thinking, "I always fail," reframing the thought to "I will learn from this," can significantly alter the emotional and behavioural outcomes.

You Are Not Your Thoughts

Thoughts are transient mental events that do not define identity or dictate actions unless we allow them to. By noticing, naming, and neutralising difficult thoughts, individuals can regain a sense of agency and make choices that align with their healing journey. Transforming limiting thought patterns into empowering ones can provide the resilience and optimism needed to navigate the challenges of addiction healing. This process, while ongoing, offers the opportunity to cultivate a more compassionate and empowered relationship with oneself.

Core Concepts

The brain constantly generates thoughts as it processes potential threats and pursues sources of pleasure.

Thoughts are neutral by nature and only gain power when engaged with. Negative thought patterns, or cognitive loops, can reinforce self-destructive behaviours if left unchecked, leading to relapse and prolonged distress.

The process of neutralising difficult thoughts involves three steps: noticing the thought, naming it to create distance, and neutralising it through questioning its helpfulness, disputing its validity, or deciding on action using a Decision-Making Matrix.

Common limiting thought patterns often involve rigid language such as "I should" or "I can't," which can reinforce feelings of guilt, shame, and helplessness. These patterns can be transformed by reframing thoughts to emphasise choice, control, and possibility.

By cultivating the skill to observe and challenge thoughts, individuals can break free from negative cycles and align their actions with their values and goals, supporting sustainable healing and personal growth.

Section 4- Building Courage

Caring For Emotions

"Your intellect may be confused, but your emotions will never lie to you." ~ *Roger Ebert*

Emotions are often seen as the enemy, with many children, especially in older generations, taught to fear, deny, repress, or avoid them. This view of emotions perceives emotions as signs of weakness, lack of discipline, or disruptions to logic and reason. Expressing emotions can lead to accusations of causing unnecessary disturbances or seeking attention. However, contemporary understanding recognises that emotions actually hold significant power and wisdom and guide people towards personal growth. Recognising and managing emotions is a critical skill in The Addiction Healing Pathway, serving as a foundation for self-compassion and enabling a more conscious and calm approach to the healing process.

Understanding and connecting with emotions is essential because emotions act as a bridge between thoughts and actions. As shown in the Cognitive Behavioural Therapy (CBT) model in the previous chapter, emotions are the drivers that spur action or inaction. Without emotional triggers, such as anger, excitement, fear, or love, human behaviour would lack motivation. Thus, listening to and correctly interpreting emotional cues is crucial to taking actions that support the healing journey and foster reconnection with one's authentic self.

What Are Emotions?

Emotions are the result of electrical signals in the brain that extend their influence throughout the body, manifesting as feelings. Their nature is captured in the word 'emotion', which can be broken down into 'e-motion,' meaning energy in motion[33]. This energy creates various reactions within the physical body, which can be intense and unsettling, or inspiring and uplifting. While some emotions generate psychological and even physical discomfort, they can also cause pronounced pleasurable sensations.

Emotions as Messengers

Emotions not only serve as a foundation for self-compassion, which is integral to the spiritual level of The Addiction Healing Pathway, but they also act as messengers of necessary steps for personal growth and learning. When we are willing to listen, our emotions can provide valuable insights, enhancing our confidence along the healing path.

According to Jim Dethmer[34], there are five primary emotions, each conveying specific messages:

Anger: Indicates that something is no longer beneficial and requires change. What needs to change could be outdated beliefs, behaviours, or relationships. It calls for establishing or reinforcing boundaries and the capacity to say "no" without justification.

Fear: Signals that something important needs to be faced or learned. It encourages full presence and awareness, prompting attention to new skills or behaviours that need to be acquired.

Sadness: Reflects the need to let go of something significant that is departing. It urges acceptance of reality and the release of roles, dreams, behaviours, or relationships that no longer serve the healing process.

Happiness: Suggests that something or someone should be celebrated or appreciated. It calls for taking the time to acknowledge personal achievements or positive experiences, fostering a sense of internal wellbeing.

Sexual Feelings: These feelings indicate a time for new ideas, creativity, and innovation. They encourage building upon these ideas and taking action to create something unique.

The 90-Second Rule

Emotions can be likened to waves, varying in duration and intensity. Some emotions resemble brief ripples, barely noticeable, while others can feel like overwhelming tsunamis. However, it has been found that the average emotional wave lasts only 90 seconds[35]. This understanding can be a powerful tool in managing emotions. While certain emotions may seem persistent, they typically dissipate within this short timeframe.

If emotions persist beyond 90 seconds, it is often due to:

- Multiple small waves occur consecutively, making it difficult to discern when one wave ends, and another begins.
- A cognitive loop, where thoughts perpetuate a cycle of difficult emotions, actions, and outcomes, thereby sustaining and intensifying the emotional experience.

This knowledge can be particularly empowering when dealing with challenging emotions such as cravings. Cravings often involve complex emotions like fear and desire, which can be experienced physically. Understanding that these intense feelings are likely to pass within 90 seconds allows individuals to employ coping mechanisms or distractions to endure the wave without succumbing to it.

Emotions of Force vs. Power

Emotions are sometimes categorised as 'good' or 'bad' based on whether they provide pleasant or unpleasant physical sensations. Dr. David Hawkins, however, offers an alternative classification in his Levels of Consciousness model, developed through Applied Kinesiology (AK) studies[36].

In this model, emotions traditionally seen as distressing, such as shame, guilt, fear, and anger, are categorised as emotions of Force. These emotions exert pressure, are life-destroying and influence behaviours either by causing inaction or demanding excessive effort. They constrain individuals, creating a sense of obligation and burden, and often lead to a feeling of being out of control of one's life and destiny.

Figure 11 - The Levels of Consciousness by Dr David Hawkins

Levels of Consciousness by Dr David Hawkins

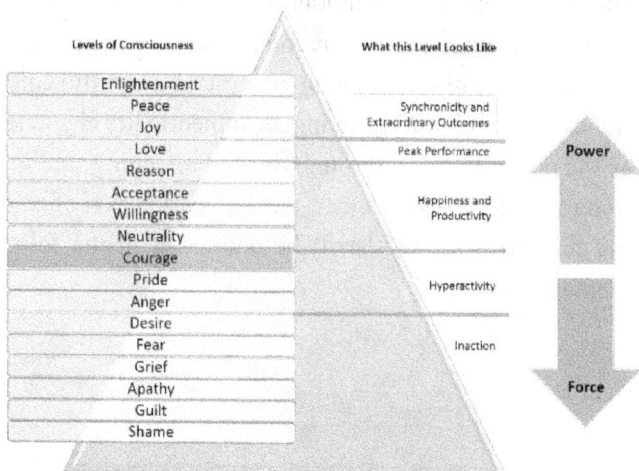

Levels of Consciousness	What this Level Looks Like
Enlightenment	
Peace	Synchronicity and Extraordinary Outcomes
Joy	
Love	Peak Performance
Reason	
Acceptance	Happiness and Productivity
Willingness	
Neutrality	
Courage	
Pride	Hyperactivity
Anger	
Desire	
Fear	Inaction
Grief	
Apathy	
Guilt	
Shame	

Power

Force

Conversely, there are emotions or states of being that draw upon intrinsic strength, are life-affirming and allow individuals to live authentically. These are known as emotions of Power and include acceptance, reason, love, joy, and peace. While Force emotions may appear undesirable compared to Power emotions, Dr. Hawkins suggests that experiencing lower-level emotions is part of a necessary journey through various states of consciousness. These emotions offer insights into personal and universal dynamics, motivating one to progress toward higher levels of consciousness. Only by experiencing the constraints of emotions like shame, guilt, anger and fear can individuals gain the motivation and skills needed to seek freedom and fulfilment.

Courage is central to the transition from Force emotions to Power emotions, acting as a bridge between these two states of existence. It is also critical in The Addiction Healing Pathway, enabling individuals to undertake the deep, reflective work required to reconnect with their true selves. It facilitates the shift from being governed by harmful emotions and external opinions to living an authentic life characterised by the power to move through these challenging states rather than to be stuck within them. Further exploration of courage, and how to achieve it, will be addressed in the following chapter.

Core Concepts

Emotions play a crucial role in guiding actions and fostering personal growth.

Emotions act as a bridge between thoughts and actions, driving behaviours that can either support or hinder the healing journey.

Emotions can be seen as "energy in motion," generating both psychological and physical responses in the body. They serve as messengers, indicating areas that require attention or change.

Emotions are transient and typically last only 90 seconds. Prolonged emotional distress often results from cognitive loops where thoughts are used to reinforce and escalate existing emotions.

Emotions can be categorised as either Force or Power. Force emotions, like shame, guilt, pride and anger, constrain and exert pressure, often leading to a sense of being overwhelmed. Power emotions, such as acceptance, love, reason and joy, draw from inner strength and promote authentic living.

Courage serves as the bridge between Force and Power emotions, enabling individuals to move from states of constraint to empowerment.

The journey through emotions, from Force to Power, is a key aspect of healing, highlighting the importance of experiencing and understanding all emotions as part of the broader process of personal growth and self-

The Process of Courage

Living at the lower levels of consciousness and operating from the emotions of Force (such as shame, guilt, fear, and anger), the world feels hopeless, miserable, and scary. But through achieving courage a person can gain a new perspective, and challenges become changes for growth.

What Is Courage?

If you look in the dictionary, you will see that the definition of courage is:

"The ability to do something that frightens one. "[37]

This definition holds the key to what courage is all about. Courage does not mean that you don't feel afraid. It is the exact opposite. Fear is an inherent part of courage. In fact, without fear, bravery does not exist. But courage is choosing to move beyond fear. It is the choice to sit with the discomfort of the unknown because of something more important.

"Courage is not the absence of fear, but rather the assessment that something else is more important than fear."
~ Franklin D. Roosevelt

To progress along the Addiction Healing Pathway, a person will need to decide that reconnecting with their true and amazing spirit is more important than allowing fear to keep them stuck in addiction. They will need to decide that stepping into their power is more valuable than giving in to their anxiety. This choice is not necessarily a discrete, single decision but an ongoing process of trying new activities, meeting new people and finding those things that facilitate the movement towards and strengthen the spirit.

Courage Is a Skill

Courage is not a quality endowed at birth or something given by our Fairy Godmother with a wave of a wand. It is an ability developed over time and with dedicated practice. Becoming courageous is just like the process of learning to read, drive, or to build big biceps. It is achieved through practice - by doing the activity and increasing the difficulty over time. Dr. Russ Harris outlines the specific steps to build courage in his model, The Confidence Cycle[38].

Figure 12 - The Confidence Cycle

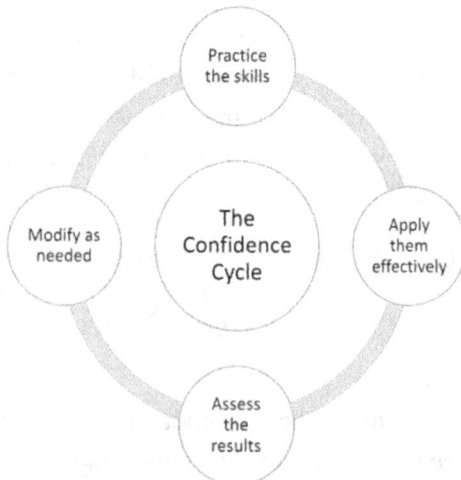

Working through these steps will build confidence in any new endeavour, be it learning to dance, speak Spanish, or live life without an addiction. More than this, though, engaging the Confidence Cycle in your daily life builds faith and trust in the ability to learn new things—that growth is possible and that are you not powerless to make change.

The Confidence Cycle also supports my passionate belief that a lapse means you are not starting all over again. As you can see, to maintain any period of abstinence or altered behaviour, a person would have worked through at least one, if not several, action cycles. The sobriety skills have been applied, even for a short time, and so much has been learnt already. As a result, there is improved intelligence about what worked with these new behaviours and what didn't. A lapse is only a failure if there is no learning from it. Otherwise, a lapse is a very valid part of the process of learning and mastery of life without a crutch.

The Actions Come First – Feelings Come Later

Notice that the Confidence Cycle above begins with the step of 'practising the skills', not with' feeling courageous.' There is a sinister belief that you have to feel confident or courageous before you do something. However, science has shown that it is the other way around. The actions of courage come first, and the feelings of courage come later.

"Hoping drains your energy. Action creates energy." ~
Robert Kiyosaki

I would go further, though and suggest that not feeling confident is absolutely expected from someone who is seeking to heal from addiction. This is because addiction is known; the person has intimate experience with the rituals and routines that go with it. In many ways, addiction is a devil, but it is the devil that is known. Moving away from addiction means entering unchartered territory and beginning something new. A new way of life is being established new parts of the self are being discovered. The old way of addiction was deadly but familiar. This new path is unknown and unfamiliar, and for this reason, it will be uncomfortable. But being uncomfortable shows that you are making change, moving away from being stuck in self-harm. In this way, discomfort is a sure sign of progress and healing, reassuring you that you are on the right path.

The Ultimate Act of Courage- Honesty

The word courage is derived from the Latin word 'cor', which means heart. It was originally used to denote that a person was speaking their full truth. This is a beautiful way of thinking about courage. One of the bravest things someone can do is be fully honest with themselves about where they are on their healing journey.

"Owning our story and loving ourselves through that process is the bravest thing we'll ever do." ~ Brené Brown

---

There can be great fear attached to admitting just how bad an addiction has become or how little progress has been made. I am certainly guilty of this. I often sat in the rehab classes putting forward my action plans to stay sober, while in the back of my mind, knowing full well I was also planning a bust.

If I had been honest to myself and the class and confessed that I was scheming to relapse, what would have happened? I don't think a bolt of lightning would have struck me through the ceiling. I think the counsellor and the other students would have rallied around me and given it their all to bolster my resolve to stay sober. I suspect that my admission would have also given others in the room permission to begin to be honest with themselves as well. Pretending that everything was OK was of no service to my healing journey. It also did not benefit anyone else in the room who may have been struggling.

"Vulnerability is not weakness; it's our greatest measure of courage". ~ Brené Brown

Do not underestimate the commitment and strength required to speak your full truth, even if it is only to yourself. Likewise, do not underestimate just how powerful this act of honesty is to your healing. The day you take off the superhero mask, you can be truly free. The day you drop the superhero cape, you can learn to fly all by yourself. And in doing so, you might also help others find their wings. Your honest vulnerability will be of greater benefit to others than your superficial strength ever will be.

Core Concepts

Courage is not the absence of fear, but the decision that something else is more important. It is the ability to face discomfort and uncertainty for the sake of something more important, such as healing from addiction and reconnecting with one's true self.

Courage is not an innate quality but a skill that can be developed through practice.

The Confidence Cycle developed by Dr Russ Harris outlines steps for building courage: practising skills, applying them effectively, assessing outcomes, and making modifications.

The Confidence Cycle shows that lapses are not failures but learning opportunities, allowing individuals to improve their approach and continue progressing.

The actions of confidence come first; the feelings of confidence come second.

The journey of healing from addiction involves discomfort because it requires moving away from familiar, albeit harmful, patterns.

Courage's ultimate expression is honesty, particularly with oneself.

Embracing honesty allows individuals to shed pretence, liberating them to live authentically, and to foster genuine connections.

Healing the Past

"I am not what happened to me; I am what I choose to become." ~ Carl Jung

Just as I was about to begin editing this chapter, I ran into a friend that I had not seen in years. This was a friend who caught me stealing beers from his fridge and from whom I nicked spare change that he left lying around to fund my next bottle of cheap wine. The feeling I had when I saw him reinforced for me that I can never 'recover' from addiction. You see sides of yourself and do things that will stick with you forever. But I can heal the wounds, allow the past to be in the past, and move forward with care and compassion for the scars.

Like the angst I felt on seeing my friend, much of the heartache we experience on the healing journey is grounded in the past. For instance, feelings of shame and guilt are caused by actions we have done that are against societal expectations. Anger indicates that our valued boundaries have been broken or that we did not get something we wanted. Pride is centred around things that we have previously gained or achieved. Even our cravings are created from and reinforced by past pleasure experiences. These past events and experiences may be long gone, yet they can still haunt us and limit our faith in ourselves and our ability to heal.

> *"Sometimes, you just have to make peace with your past to keep your future from becoming a constant battle." ~ Susan Gale*

This is not to say we justify or condone anything that we have done in the past. We cannot just sweep things away and pretend they did not happen. But neither can we keep them as weights around our necks like some symbol of repentance or self-imposed punishment. Self-flagellation is of no service to anyone. What is done is done. You cannot change it. The most important thing you need to do now is learn from it. And the most important action you will ever take is what you choose to do next with what you have learnt.

Counter-Productive Shortcuts

Two common yet counter-productive shortcuts that individuals often take in dealing with past trauma are:

1. Blaming others
2. Wallowing in shame and guilt.

While these approaches may offer some immediate relief, they ultimately undermine the development of courage and self-acceptance.

Blaming Others

> *"You can fail many times, but you are not a failure until you begin to blame somebody else." ~ John Burroughs.*

Blaming others for past actions or current situations can initially feel satisfying, as it allows for the deflection of responsibility and accountability. This approach can create a false sense of relief by building a narrative that places the blame entirely on external factors, thereby avoiding the need for self-reflection and personal growth.

For example, in a situation where a friend catches another in the act of stealing, it is easy to construct a narrative where the friend's perceived parental negligence or peer pressure is blamed for the individual's actions. However, this mindset also relinquishes personal power, suggesting that external forces control one's life. While this may provide short-term satisfaction, it creates a barrier to self-growth and prevents individuals from focusing on their potential and purpose.

Wallowing in Shame and Guilt

Shame and guilt are known as the sister emotions. They are similar in that they take up the lowest sections of the Level of Consciousness, suggesting they have the potential to impact a person most negatively. While these terms are often used interchangeably, they have different connotations. Shame says that I am a bad person and do not deserve to be within the tribe. Guilt says that I have done something bad, and must now seek to make amends.

Both emotions are situated at the bottom of the Levels of Consciousness model and as such contain the potential to impact a person negatively. They act as a force upon a person and can lead to inaction and keeping a person stuck in unhelpful patterns of behaviour. When prolonged, these emotions can foster a sense of unworthiness and self-hatred, which are counter-productive to the healing process. Instead of serving as a catalyst for positive change, persistent shame and guilt can reinforce negative self-perceptions, obstructing the journey towards self-acceptance and self-compassion.

A common challenge in this context is the expectation—whether self-imposed or from others—that a display of repentance is necessary to demonstrate understanding and remorse for past actions. While the desire to express regret and accountability is valid, it is crucial to differentiate between constructive reflection and self-imposed punishment. Those who genuinely care will not demand prolonged suffering as a sign of repentance; they will support efforts to move forward and grow.

The Road Less Travelled: The 4 R's

An alternative to blame, shame, and guilt involves the following four steps, referred to as the 4 R's:

1. Respect
2. Regret
3. Responsibility
4. Restoration.

These steps draw from Buddhist teachings on the opponent powers, which focus on purifying the negative imprints made from harmful actions and restoring mental balance so that one can move forward positively[39].

Respect

Respect involves acknowledging the value and lessons that emerge from past challenges. While it may be difficult to respect the hardships endured, they have contributed to the current state of resilience and progress. Respect entails recognising the strength developed through these experiences and celebrating the perseverance demonstrated in overcoming them.

This step also includes acknowledging that for every negative emotion encountered, there exists an opportunity to learn about its positive counterpart. Navigating grief may help one gain a deeper understanding of love; confronting shame can teach one the value of self-acceptance. Respecting the past means valuing these insights and the strength they have cultivated.

Respect also means giving due regard to the others involved in the situation, and their needs to feel safe, heard, validated and to have the space and time for their own processing of the events and their impact. This is important as each person involved will have their own journey through the healing process.

Regret

Regret serves as a constructive alternative to guilt. It provides a forward-looking approach that acknowledges the harm caused while seeking opportunities for healing and growth. Unlike guilt, which often leads to self-reproach and stagnation, regret facilitates a more mature and positive response to past mistakes.

Regret requires an honest and comprehensive reflection on the impact of one's actions. This step goes beyond superficial acknowledgment and calls for a full understanding of the harm caused, allowing for meaningful learning and transformation.

Responsibility

Responsibility involves recognising one's role in past actions and the capacity to shape the future. Rather than assigning blame to external factors, responsibility emphasises taking proactive steps to alter one's circumstances. Such actions might involve:

- Accepting one's role in the harm
- Distancing oneself from negative influences
- Making amends where possible
- Seeking assistance to prevent the same situation being repeated.

Responsibility is an active process that shifts the focus from judgment to positive change.

Restoration

Restoration encompasses two key aspects: rebuilding trust in oneself and repairing relationships with others.

Restoring Faith in Oneself

Throughout the course of addiction, a tragedy occurs, and this is that a person loses trust in themselves. They lose faith that they are able to care for those that they profess to love, and to make the right decisions for their own wellbeing. Self-trust is eroded by repeated harmful actions. However, the same way that faith in oneself has been lost, it can be restored. Just as trust was eroded by making bad decisions over and over again, it can be regained by repeatedly no making good decisions. You only get trust by doing the same right action over and over and over again.

Restoring Relationships with Others

Similarly, restoring trust with others is a product of hard work. It is the result of action. Trust is the culmination of the countless small decisions and tiny actions you take every day. The people around you also have many wounds, and so they will not be willing to hand trust over to you without further thought. Trust is something you earn back from them by consistent effort.

Restoring relationships with others also involves making amends for past actions where possible. This process requires time, patience, and a willingness to engage with those affected. It is important to recognise that healing relationships may take longer for others than it does for oneself, as those hurt may still carry the trauma of past experiences. You cannot dictate how a person may respond, or whether they will ever be willing to receive your apology, but you can control the respect and regard in which you hold their experiences.

For it may be the case that those affected are not ready or willing to forgive. In such cases, the focus should remain on personal accountability and learning rather than being dependent on others' responses.

You can find more about the process of rebuilding trust later in this book.

Moving Forward

The influence of past events on one's life can be profound, often perpetuating guilt, shame, and self-reproach. However, time is a finite resource, and how it is spent can significantly impact one's journey. The choice lies between remaining anchored to past mistakes or embracing a path of respect, regret, responsibility, and restoration. The former may lead to continued self-sabotage, while the latter offers the possibility of healing and freedom.

"You are not your past. Although you are changed and shaped by past experiences, who you were yesterday does not control the person you have the potential to become tomorrow." ~ Sue Augustine

---

Core Concepts

Healing from addiction often involves confronting the past, where feelings of shame, guilt, anger, and cravings are rooted in previous actions.

Making peace with the past does not mean condoning harmful actions or ignoring their impact. Instead, it involves acknowledging that the past cannot be changed and focusing on learning.

Blaming others and wallowing in shame and guilt are counter-productive shortcuts. Blaming deflects responsibility. Prolonged shame and guilt can lead to self-hatred and obstruct the healing process.

The 4 R's—Respect, Regret, Responsibility, and Restoration—offer a constructive path forward:

Respect: Recognise the value and lessons learned from past challenges and respect the other person's experiences and healing process.

Regret: Embrace regret as a forward-looking alternative to guilt, focusing on learning from mistakes and seeking positive change.

Responsibility: Take accountability for past actions and recognise the ability to shape the future.

Restoration: Focus on rebuilding self-trust and restoring relationships with others through taking consistent helpful action.

Section 5- Connecting With Spirit

Connecting with Spirit

"To be yourself in a world that is constantly trying to make you something else is the greatest accomplishment." ~ Ralph Waldo Emerson

This chapter represents a pivotal moment in The Addiction Healing Pathway. Every preceding step has led to this critical juncture: reconnecting with one's true self or spirit. This reconnection aims to foster a sense of understanding and acceptance of the self, which can then be extended outwardly to engage with the world in a meaningful way.

The disconnection from the spirit is what allows addiction to take root and persist. Like a parasite that thrives in a weakened host, addiction exploits the gaps left by a fractured sense of self. While cognitive and emotional vulnerabilities certainly play roles, the underlying disconnect from the spirit is a foundational issue that needs addressing. This stage of The Addiction Healing Pathway emphasises healing this wound by rediscovering and nurturing the unique and intrinsic qualities that define the individual.

Distinguishing Between Who You Are and What You Do

A crucial aspect of this stage is distinguishing between "who you are" and "what you do." Although repeated actions influence how others perceive an individual and can shape one's character, they do not necessarily represent the core of who that person is. Misconstruing actions with identity can create a significant barrier to healing, as individuals may struggle to forgive themselves for past behaviours that do not align with their true selves.

During addiction, individuals often engage in behaviours that are incongruent with their core values and self-concept. It is important to recognise that while the individual carried out these actions, they were driven by the complexities of addiction and do not necessarily reflect the true nature of the person. Understanding this distinction can be pivotal in fostering self-compassion and advancing along the path of healing.

As we have heard, addictions fulfil specific emotional needs, such as alleviating the pain of not living authentically, managing the internal conflict with one's spirit, or addressing the desire to reach one's full potential. Addiction may temporarily offer relief or fulfilment of these needs, but it fails to provide sustainable solutions. Only through reconnecting with the spirit can one establish a stable and enduring source of inner strength and resilience, capable of withstanding life's challenges.

Defining the Spirit

Understanding the concept of the spirit is essential before exploring how to reconnect with it. Definitions of the spirit can vary widely, influenced by personal beliefs, upbringing, and religious or cultural contexts. For the purposes of this discussion, the spirit is the unique set of values, passions, and aspirations that an individual brings into the world, along with the distinct ways in which these are expressed.

The word spirit may be troublesome for some people, so here are some other similar terms that you may be more comfortable with:

- Essence
- A sense of purpose
- Meaning
- The power within
- Innermost self
- Vibe
- Mojo
- Energy.

The thing about spirit is that there is not one part of a person's physical being in which it resides. It has no tangible boundaries. It not only delivers peace and love for where we are right now but calls us to be more, to develop, to learn and to grow. It holds us safely where we are but also encourages us to embrace this adventure called life.

What Does Connection with Spirit Feel Like?

Connection with the spirit is often characterised by feelings of inner balance, purpose, and inspiration. Wayne Dyer describes this state as being accompanied by strong emotions such as passion and bliss, which indicate alignment with one's true self.

"Strong emotions such as passion and bliss are indications that you're connected to Spirit, or inspired,' if you will."

In this state, individuals are more likely to experience positive outcomes and a sense of fulfilment as they engage with the world in meaningful ways.

It is important to note that connection with the spirit does not imply a life devoid of challenges or negative emotions. Rather, it involves having a guiding sense of purpose that helps individuals remain anchored and inspired, even when faced with difficulties. When connected with the spirit, individuals are better equipped to manage life's ups and downs, drawing on their inner resources to maintain a sense of direction and wellbeing.

The Consequences of Disconnection

The consequences of disconnection from the spirit are often manifested in the behaviours and experiences associated with addiction. This disconnection can lead to a range of cognitive, emotional, and physical symptoms that exacerbate the challenges of addiction and healing. The primary consequence, however, is the sense of regret that may emerge at the end of life when individuals reflect on missed opportunities to live authentically and fully.

Bronnie Ware, a palliative care nurse, documented the most common regrets of those nearing the end of their lives. She wanted to know their greatest regrets and what they would do differently with a second chance at life. While these conversations were heartbreaking, they provide such wisdom and a gift for us to learn from. Here are the top five regrets from those who were dying[40]:

- I wish I pursued my dreams and aspirations and not the life others expected of me.
- I wish I did not work so hard.
- I wish I dared to express my feelings and speak my mind.
- I wish I had stayed in touch with my friends.
- I wish I had let myself be happier.

These reflections serve as a powerful reminder of the importance of reconnecting with the spirit and making choices that are true to oneself. The desire to live authentically and to pursue one's unique potential is a central theme in the accounts of those nearing the end of life. By reconnecting with the spirit, individuals can mitigate the risk of regret and ensure that their lives are guided by their deepest values and aspirations.

Reconnecting with Spirit

So how do you work to find your spirit? It comes down to finding a balance between:

- Listening; and
- Taking action.

You need to be still, quiet, listen for the calls of the spirit, know when you are close, and know if you have moved further away.

Then in between the listening, you need to dig. You need to take action, do things, experiment to see if this will move you closer. And then, after a period of action, you need to stop again and listen.

And so the journey to reconnect with the spirit is an interplay between action and stillness, progress and peace, stimulation and silence and expedition and retreat. Without action and experimenting, you won't know what may work for you and what inspires you. Likewise, without taking some time to be still and listen, you miss out on the important messages that your spirit is sending about where to go next.

In this way, spirituality then is the practice of reconnecting and maintaining the connection with your spirit. We do things to find what is meaningful for us and how we want to express it in this world. Just as we care for our bodies, thoughts and emotions, spirituality is the process of caring for our spirit and allowing it to live openly and fully.

Techniques for Listening to the Spirit

Some of the best instructions I have found on how to listen come from Tibetan Buddhism. Here it is taught that there are three precious pills that act as the medicine for listening fully[41]. These pills are:

1. Stillness
2. Silence
3. Spaciousness

By sitting, standing or lying still, you give your brain a break from processing all of the data you create when you move. It removes the first layer of physical distractions and allows you to move deeper into thoughts and emotions.

Concentrating on the silence around you is an incredibly effective way to bring silence into your internal world. Learning to become aware of the quiet helps you find the gaps between thoughts and feelings and reinforces the transient nature of both. This makes it much easier to let go of those that trouble you and prevent clinging to those that make you feel good.

When we are operating from shame, fear, guilt or pride, our world can feel very small. To counter this, the final pill of spaciousness calls on us to become aware of the great space around us and within us. If you are outside, look up to the sky. Witness the expansive freedom that abounds on our planet and within our universe. Then you may be able to bring this view inwards and see if you can get a sense of just how vast and limitless your potential is.

Being still, silent and aware of the spaciousness is the way we listen to our spirit. It is a skilful way to help you come to know that:

"You are the sky. Everything else is just the weather." ~ *Pema Chodron*

You may be thinking that this technique is very similar to meditation, and you are absolutely right. The 3-pill technique is a meditation that you can use at any time, for any length of time when you need to regroup and reconnect. Many other meditation techniques are wonderful aids to help you listen to your true nature.

Notice, though, that none of these descriptions of being connected with the spirit suggests that this state is devoid of any problems, concerns, sadness or 'muck' of modern-day life. What they do suggest, though, is that when you are connected with the spirit:

- Your sense of purpose grounds you in what is truly important and inspires you to keep going.
- You are comfortable in your skin and flexible enough to move through or around obstacles as they arise.

The ancient Tibetan practice of soul retrieval suggests that connection with the spirit shows up as a balance of the five elements:

1. Earth – grounded and connected
2. Air – flexible and moving
3. Fire – full of joy and inspiration
4. Water – comfortable and fluid
5. Space – open and accommodating.

When you are settled in stillness, silence and spaciousness, it is an opportune moment to investigate the presence of the five elements within your body and mind. You can check in with each of these by asking yourself the following questions, and then listen closely for the response:

1. Earth – am I feeling grounded, balanced and connected?
2. Air – am I flexible and able to move freely in body and mind?
3. Fire – am I full of joy and inspiration?
4. Water – do I feel comfortable in my skin and able to navigate calmly around obstacles?
5. Space – do I feel open and accommodating to the people and experiences that come my way?

If any elements feel stuck or stagnant, you can move to the next stage of reconnection – taking action.

Taking Action to Reconnect with the Spirit

In addition to listening, reconnecting with the spirit requires taking purposeful action. Action serves as a means of testing alignment with the spirit and allows individuals to experiment with different approaches to living authentically. It is important to approach this process with a mindset of curiosity and openness, viewing each action as an opportunity to learn and grow.

The focus should be on taking small, deliberate steps rather than attempting large-scale changes all at once. Individuals can gradually build confidence and adjust as needed by engaging in manageable actions and observing their effects. This iterative process, often referred to as the Confidence Cycle, involves practising skills, evaluating results, and refining actions to better align with one's values and goals.

Living by Values

Identifying and living by personal values is a practical way to deepen the connection with the spirit. Values represent the principles and behaviours that are most meaningful and guide decision-making. By clarifying core values, individuals can create a framework for making choices that are consistent with their true selves.

To identify values, individuals may consider what they want to be known for and what qualities they wish to embody. Reflecting on these values and assessing how well they are being lived out can provide a roadmap for personal growth and action. For values that require more attention, individuals can identify specific steps to bring these values more fully into their lives, creating a series of experiments to explore through the Confidence Cycle.

A Personal and Ongoing Process

Reconnecting with the spirit is a deeply personal and ongoing process that involves both introspection and action. Individuals can cultivate a sense of authenticity and purpose by engaging in practices that foster self-awareness and alignment with personal values. This connection with the spirit provides a foundation of resilience and strength, supporting individuals as they navigate the challenges of addiction healing and beyond.

Living in alignment with the spirit is not without its challenges, as it requires a commitment to personal growth and a willingness to confront discomfort. However, the rewards of this journey are substantial, offering a sense of liberation, fulfilment, and peace. As individuals reconnect with their true selves, they can live more fully and share their unique gifts with the world.

Core Concepts

Reconnecting with the spirit addresses the root cause of addiction, laying the groundwork for a new future.

It's essential to separate actions from identity, as behaviours in addiction do not define one's core self.

The spirit represents an individual's unique values, passions, and aspirations. Connecting with it aligns actions with true nature, providing inner strength and resilience.

Disconnection from the spirit can lead to regret over unfulfilled potential and missed opportunities in life.

Reconnecting involves both:
1. Listening (through stillness, silence, spaciousness) and
2. Action (experimenting with steps aligned with personal values).

Identifying and living by values guides authentic actions and deepens the connection with the spirit, helping align life with one's true self.

Reconnecting with the spirit is an ongoing journey requiring introspection and continual questioning.

Being True to Something Bigger Than You

"Life asks of every individual a contribution, and it is up to that individual to discover what it should be." — Viktor E. Frankl

Reconnecting with, appreciating, and celebrating your unique spirit is crucial in healing from addiction. Understanding and embracing your distinctive and exceptional nature can address the emotional voids formed over years of neglect and establish a solid foundation for a life filled with love and joy. It might seem like the journey ends once you have reconnected with your spirit, leaving you to bask in the glow of authenticity. However, even at this stage, there is more work to be done for two main reasons:

The Continuous Process of Self-Discovery: Understanding your spirit is an ongoing journey. The world offers countless experiences, each providing an opportunity to engage intentionally, learn, and grow. Every action and interaction allow you to explore what heals and what hurts, fostering wisdom and compassion. The depth of your understanding of your spirit is limited only by your commitment to living with curiosity and an open heart and mind.

Connecting to Something Greater: Our desire to live true to our purpose can be used for more than just self-satisfaction. Humans are naturally inclined to connect with and contribute to something larger than themselves. This desire can manifest in various ways, from small acts of kindness to larger commitments to communities or causes. The concept of contributing to something greater is illustrated in Buddhism's Mahayana school, where practitioners seek enlightenment not just for their own satisfaction, but to help liberate all beings. They recognise that while personal healing is important, it is not an end in itself, but can be a conduit to greater fulfilment, as noted by Tony Robbins:

"Only those who have learned the power of sincere and selfless contribution experience life's deepest joy: true fulfilment." — *Tony Robbins*

The Impact of Contribution on Wellbeing

Numerous studies have demonstrated the importance of connection and contribution to overall wellbeing. One extensive study involving over 25,000 young adults across 58 countries found that intrinsic values, such as meaningful social connections and contributing to the community, were stronger predictors of wellbeing than extrinsic motivators like power and financial gain[42]. This research shows that our sense of contentment is deeply connected to how we engage with the world around us.

The Ripple Effect of Personal Change

We are born with unique perspectives and abilities that can enrich not only our own lives but also the lives of others. Our ability to improve our own and others' live does not necessarily require taking on roles like activism or volunteering on the front lines of global crises. Rather, it begins with small, personal changes that ripple outward, influencing those around us in subtle but significant ways. Viktor Frankl emphasised the personal nature of contribution, suggesting that life's challenge is to discover how our unique spirit can make a difference.

In the book *Active Hope*[43], Macy and Johnstone describe four levels of community through which our contributions can have an impact:

The Four Levels of Community

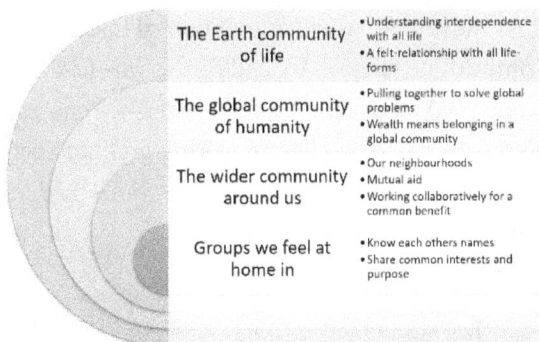

The Earth community of life	• Understanding interdependence with all life • A felt-relationship with all life-forms
The global community of humanity	• Pulling together to solve global problems • Wealth means belonging in a global community
The wider community around us	• Our neighbourhoods • Mutual aid • Working collaboratively for a common benefit
Groups we feel at home in	• Know each others names • Share common interests and purpose

Adapted from Macy, J., & Johnstone, C. (2012). *Active Hope: How to Face the Mess We're in without Going Crazy* (58069th ed.). New World Library.

Groups We Feel at Home In: These include family, close friends, religious communities, or interest groups where values and goals are shared, and individuals are known personally.

The Wider Community: This encompasses broader communities such as neighbourhoods, towns, and even national groups. It also includes clubs and volunteer organisations where people unite for a common cause.

The Global Community of Humanity: Beyond local or national boundaries, this level involves contributing to the welfare of all humans, addressing global issues that affect everyone regardless of race, religion, or nationality.

The Earth Community of Life: This level recognises the interconnectedness of all life, extending our sense of responsibility beyond humans to include all living beings and ecosystems.

As illustrated, whether your contributions remain within your immediate circle or extend further, the positive impact has the potential to spread. Acts of kindness, generosity, and support create a chain reaction, fostering gratitude and optimism that can transcend individual interactions and influence wider social circles.

"You cannot get through a single day without having an impact on the world around you. What you do makes a difference, and you have to decide what kind of a difference you want to make." — Jane Goodall

---

The Concept of a Higher Being

The model of community contribution might seem limited to Earth and humanity, but many people find meaning in connecting with concepts beyond the physical world, such as higher beings, deities, or even the broader universe. Some people may place faith in what they know as God, others in what they call the Universe, while for some, they have a broader commitment to serve their Community. While the target of connection can differ, the fundamental aspect is aligning your spirit with something greater, whether that is framed within religious, spiritual, or philosophical contexts.

Embracing Your Role in the Larger Whole

Connection to something larger than oneself can begin on a very personal level and expand outward. It's about recognising the power of even the smallest actions and their potential to inspire and affect change. This mindset helps shift the focus from self-centred healing to a broader understanding of one's role in the larger community, whether that community is local, global, or cosmic.

Being true to something bigger than oneself does not mean sacrificing personal wellbeing or neglecting individual needs. Instead, it integrates personal growth with a sense of shared purpose and responsibility. This balanced approach not only enhances individual healing but also contributes to a greater collective good. As you continue along the Addiction Healing Pathway, remember that every action, no matter how small, has the potential to make a meaningful difference.

Core Concepts

Reconnecting with your spirit is vital for healing from addiction, but the journey doesn't end there. We are called to:

- Embark on an ongoing process of self-discovery
- Connect with something greater than ourselves.

Humans naturally seek connection and contribution beyond themselves, which can bring deep joy and a sense of great fulfilment.

Studies show that meaningful connections and contributions are stronger predictors of wellbeing than external achievements like wealth or power.

Personal change creates a ripple effect, positively impacting others and extending through various levels of community, from close circles to the global and even ecological community.

Contribution doesn't have to be grand; small, personal actions can significantly influence others and foster a sense of fulfilment and shared purpose.

Being true to something bigger than yourself integrates personal growth with a sense of shared purpose and responsibility, enhancing both individual healing and collective wellbeing.

Section 6- Creating a Supportive Environment

Creating A Nurturing Environment

"Energy is contagious, positive and negative alike. I will forever be mindful of what and who I am allowing into my space." — Alex Elle.

As individuals seeking wellbeing, our physical and social environments play a critical role; they can either help or hinder our healing. Therefore, just as we pay attention to our breath, movement, medication and nutrition, we also have the ability to actively managing our surroundings to provide support for our journey.

This chapter explores two key aspects of creating a nurturing environment:

1. Physical Environment: The impact of the structures and spaces we inhabit.
2. Social Environment: The influence of the people we interact with.

Physical Environment

We are sensory beings, and we take in a great deal of information from our physical environments. What we see, hear and touch and smell can either make us feel comfortable and confident, or put us in a place of insecurity and threat. Therefore, the physical environment is a crucial factor in influencing wellbeing.

There are many variables in our surroundings that we can work with to create a nurturing and supportive physical environment. These include:

- **Sunlight:** Regular exposure to natural light has been shown to improve mood and mental health.
- **Fresh Air:** Adequate ventilation and access to clean air help invigorate the body and mind.
- **Nature:** With its calming and restorative effect, nature plays a significant role in the healing process. Whether through direct exposure or indoor plants, incorporating elements of nature can provide a much-needed respite.
- **Colour:** Surrounding oneself with uplifting colours and supportive of mental and emotional states can positively influence mood.
- **Noise:** Minimising both acute and chronic noise can reduce stress levels and improve concentration.
- **Clutter:** Keeping spaces free of unnecessary physical and digital clutter promotes a sense of order and calm.

Additionally, considering the balance of the five elements—Earth, Air, Fire, Water, and Space—can also provide a framework by which the environment can be shaped to deliver either stimulus or serenity:

- **Earth:** Incorporating natural materials or plants can foster a sense of grounding and connection to the natural world.
- **Air:** Ensuring good airflow through open windows or fans can replicate the invigorating qualities of wind.

- **Fire:** Using warm lighting or candles can bring the energising and inspirational qualities associated with sunlight.
- **Water:** Engaging with water through showers, baths, or even visual representations can evoke feelings of flexibility and resilience.
- **Space:** Creating spaciousness through decluttering or visualising open landscapes helps tap into a sense of openness and freedom.

Enhancing or subduing these elements allows for the shifting of a space to support whatever is required in the moment, be it more energy or more calm.

Social Environment

"Be careful the friends you choose, for you will become like them." — W. Clement Stone

Research, including a 30-year longitudinal study, has demonstrated that social networks significantly impact various aspects of physical health, including addictive behaviours. For example, having friends who smoke increases the likelihood of smoking by 61%. This influence extends beyond immediate contacts; even the habits of friends of friends can indirectly affect personal behaviour.

The positive aspect of this influence is that beneficial behaviours and mental states are also contagious. Happiness, for instance, can spread through social networks. A close friend's happiness increases the likelihood of being happy by 25%, and even a happy next-door neighbour can have a positive impact[44].

The message from this research is clear, choose your companions on the healing journey wisely, for they could keep you stuck in self-harm. Conversely, being surrounded by individuals who practice self-compassion and strive for personal growth can significantly support the healing journey.

Identifying Unhelpful Relationships

It is likely through addiction that you have established some unhelpful relationships. These often emerge during periods of vulnerability, and arise from people seeking solace in those also undertaking a path of self-destruction, or who appear stronger than themselves in some way. Recognising such relationships and distancing from negative influences can be challenging, but here are some sure signs that the relationship you are involved in is unhelpful:

- **Jealousy and Criticism**: Individuals who diminish accomplishments often operate from fear and insecurity. They may struggle with another's healing process, not out of malice but because it highlights their inadequacies.
- **Constant Judgment**: Relationships characterised by excessive expectations and judgment can undermine self-acceptance. When constantly evaluated or criticised, it becomes difficult to cultivate self-compassion, which is crucial for healing.

- **One-Sided Caring**: Some relationships may feel unbalanced, with one party always seeking support without reciprocating. While it may feel good to help someone initially, the lack of mutual support can become draining and unsustainable over time.
- **Negative Energy**: Frequent exposure to negative emotions like guilt, shame, fear, or anger can affect overall mood and energy levels, potentially triggering stress responses, starting downward spirals, and making it harder to stay on the path to healing.

Challenges in Leaving Unhelpful Relationships

Ending unhelpful relationships is often easier said than done and can be complicated by factors such as:

- **Sense of Obligation**: Feelings of responsibility, whether as a caregiver or due to past support received, can create a sense of duty to maintain the relationship.
- **Lack of Alternatives**: Perceived lack of options or fear of loneliness may lead to staying in a detrimental relationship.
- **Community and Belonging**: Even toxic relationships can provide a sense of belonging, which is preferable to the uncertainty of facing things alone.

Options for Addressing Unhelpful Relationships

Five options are available when dealing with unhelpful relationships, ranging from minimal intervention to more decisive actions. These include:

1. **Do Nothing**: This option is suitable if the relationship is naturally fading or insignificant. However, choosing to do something may also mean opportunities to develop courage and resilience in handling difficult relationships.

2. **Discuss Concerns**: Open communication can reveal whether the relationship is worth saving. Using respectful and assertive communication techniques, such as stating, "When you... I feel...," can help address issues. Professional assistance, like counselling or mediation, may also be beneficial in challenging conversations.

3. **Set Boundaries**: Establishing boundaries ensures both parties understand acceptable behaviours within the relationship. Communicate that criticism or harmful statements will not be tolerated, and if such behaviour continues, be prepared to leave the situation.

4. **Detachment**: Detachment involves refusing to engage with negative behaviours or emotions. Even when physically present, psychological distancing can protect from the harmful effects of the relationship.

5. **Ending the Relationship**: If other strategies fail, ending the relationship may be necessary. While this decision may involve a sense of loss, it also opens space for new, healthier connections to support personal growth and wellbeing.

Characteristics of Supportive Relationships

In the early stages of healing, it can be difficult to trust those offering help, especially if there is uncertainty about committing to change. For example, I remember calling my psychiatrist a dictator because I felt he was treating me like a child and trying to control my life. Now I can honestly say that he saved my life. That is why I think it is important to have a checklist of the characteristics of a helpful relationship. This way, if you are unsure about whether the help you are receiving is right for you, you have some criteria to judge it by. Even though you may not trust this person yet, they are likely working in your best interests when they[45]:

- **Encourage Self-Acceptance and Compassion**: Supportive individuals celebrate successes and promote self-compassion during setbacks. They encourage self-love, regardless of circumstances.
- **Promote Honesty**: True supporters hold individuals accountable and encourage integrity, even when it involves difficult conversations. They help maintain high moral standards and align actions with personal values and goals.
- **Are Present**: Supportive people offer their full attention, listen actively, and validate feelings. They are genuine in their interest in understanding the individual's physical, mental, and emotional state.
- **Inspire Positive Change**: Supportive individuals inspire others to reach their potential by serving as role models through their commitment, kindness, and persistence. They encourage others to continue striving, even after setbacks.

Creating a physically and socially nurturing environment provides a foundation for sustained long-term healing. We have the ability to bring greater consciousness and care to both our surroundings and relationships, and have these essential elements of our environment become sources of support and sustenance on the healing pathway.

Core Concepts

Your physical and social environments can either help or hinder your healing journey.

A nurturing physical environment enhances healing through elements like sunlight, fresh air, nature, uplifting colours, reduced noise, and minimal clutter. Considering the five elements—Earth, Air, Fire, Water, and Space—further allows you to tailor a space to support either stimulation or serenity.

Social environments significantly impact behaviour and wellbeing. Surrounding yourself with positive, supportive individuals can encourage healthy habits.

Options for dealing with unhelpful relationships range from doing nothing, discussing concerns, setting boundaries, detaching emotionally, to ending the relationship.

Supportive relationships are characterised by encouragement of self-acceptance, honesty, presence, and inspiration towards positive change. They validate your journey and hold you accountable in a compassionate way.

Creating a nurturing environment through positive physical and social influences lays a strong foundation for ongoing healing, resilience, and personal growth.

A Word on Enabling Relationships

"The best way to move forward is to let go of the people holding you back." ~ Anonymous

One of the most complex and challenging dynamics, particularly in the early stages of healing, involves relationships with enablers—those who consciously or unconsciously support self-destructive behaviours. In the context of addiction, an enabler is someone who facilitates the continued use of addictive substances or the continuation of addictive activities.

Enablers are not always individuals who overtly encourage addictive behaviours; their actions can be subtle and even appear as kindness or assistance. Subtle sabotage can make recognising enablers particularly difficult, as it often masquerades under the guise of care or support.

The Enabling Continuum

Enablers can vary significantly in their manifestations, ranging from passive indifference to active encouragement. The following descriptions illustrate a continuum of enabling behaviours, from the most passive to the most overt.

Ignorers

The most passive form of enabling involves ignoring the presence of substance use or addictive behaviours. Adopting an "ignorance is bliss" philosophy, this type of enabler may believe that the addiction is merely a phase. Alternatively, the individual may feel overwhelmed or powerless to intervene, leading them to ignore the situation as a means of self-protection.

Figure 14 - Types of Enabling Behaviours

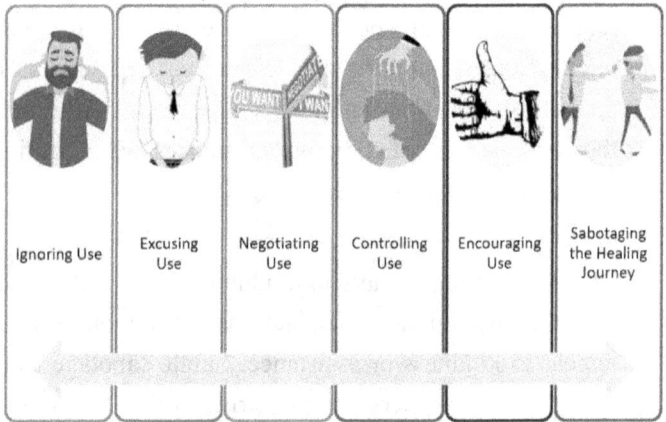

| Ignoring Use | Excusing Use | Negotiating Use | Controlling Use | Encouraging Use | Sabotaging the Healing Journey |

Excusers

Excusers move beyond passive ignorance by rationalising addictive behaviour. They might justify excessive drinking, drug use, or compulsive activities as coping mechanisms for stress or personal hardship. They may also dismiss the behaviour as typical or excusable, thus perpetuating the cycle of addiction without direct confrontation.

Negotiators

Negotiators attempt to set boundaries on addictive behaviour, often through agreements or compromises. They may allow certain behaviours under specific conditions, such as drinking only after a certain time or engaging in addictive activity only on weekends. While this approach might seem like a step toward control, it reinforces the idea that the behaviour is acceptable under certain circumstances.

Controllers

When negotiation fails, some enablers may take on a more controlling role, restricting access to money, substances, or activities in an attempt to manage the addiction. This controlling behaviour is often well-intentioned, stemming from a desire to help the person struggling with addiction. However, it maintains the dynamic of the enabler holding power over the addicted individual, often leading to further conflict.

Encouragers

Encouragers actively support the addiction by downplaying the consequences of the behaviour or by glorifying the perceived benefits of the substance or activity. They may discourage the pursuit of healing by emphasising the discomforts of withdrawal or suggesting that the person is more likable or functional when using. Encouragers may also challenge the individual to participate in addictive behaviours as a means of maintaining social or relational ties.

Saboteurs

At the most extreme end of the continuum are saboteurs, who deliberately create situations that increase the likelihood of relapse. They may manufacture stress or conflict to provoke a return to addictive behaviours, positioning themselves as the provider of the substance or activity as a solution. This behaviour is highly manipulative and harmful, as it not only undermines healing but actively works against it.

The Impact of Enabling Behaviours

None of these enabling behaviours facilitates healing; rather, they perpetuate the cycle of addiction and often place the enabler in a position of control. Even those enablers who act out of concern may inadvertently undermine the trust, openness, and honesty necessary for healing.

Enabling Is About the Enabler

It is important to recognise that enabling behaviours often reflect the enabler's own insecurities and fears rather than the needs of the person with the addiction. For example, enablers may fear losing their own vices if they confront someone else's addiction or worry about the changes that sobriety might bring to their relationship dynamics. These fears can manifest in various ways, such as:

- Rationalising their own harmful habits by pointing to the addict's behaviour.
- Fearing rejection or abandonment if they confront the addictive behaviour.
- Avoiding conflict with family members or other authorities who disapprove of the addict's behaviour.

- Fearing a loss of purpose or control if the addicted individual no longer relies on them.

These fears and the resulting enabling behaviours represent attempts to control a situation that feels chaotic and unmanageable. However, they do not contribute to a healthy, sustainable relationship and instead keep both parties stuck in self-harm.

The Evolution of Enabling Roles Over Time

Enabling behaviours are not static; they can evolve as the addiction progresses. Understanding these potential transitions can help you prepare for changes in your relationships.

From Excuser to Controller

As addiction escalates, passive excuses may no longer suffice. The enabler might first attempt to negotiate limits on the behaviour, but as these agreements fail, they may resort to control measures. This shift is often driven by a realisation that the addiction is spiralling and that stricter actions are necessary. While the intent may be to help, this dynamic often results in a policing role that strains the relationship.

From Encourager to Saboteur

For some enablers, the prospect of the individual overcoming addiction poses a threat to their sense of security or purpose. As a result, they may transition from subtly encouraging the behaviour to actively sabotaging healing efforts. This evolution is often driven by deep-seated fears of losing the role or connection that the addiction maintains.

Self-Enabling: A Critical Reflection

A challenging aspect of dealing with enabling behaviours is recognising when these actions are self-directed. Many individuals struggling with addiction may unconsciously enable their own behaviours, whether by ignoring the severity of their actions, excusing lapses, attempting to negotiate use, or actively sabotaging healing efforts. This internal conflict can be more difficult to address than external relationships, as it requires an ongoing commitment to self-awareness and accountability.

Ultimately, understanding the dynamics of enablement— whether they come from others or from within—is a critical step in breaking free from the cycle of addiction. Acknowledging and addressing these influences can foster a healthier, more supportive environment conducive to long-term healing.

Core Concepts

Enablers are individuals who, knowingly or unknowingly, support self-destructive behaviours in someone with an addiction.

Enabling behaviours fall on a continuum:
- Ignorers: Ignore the addiction, believing it's a phase or feeling powerless to intervene.
- Excusers: Justify the behaviour as a coping mechanism or normalise it.
- Negotiators: Set conditions for the addictive behaviour, inadvertently accepting it under certain terms.
- Controllers: Try to restrict access to substances or activities, which can lead to power struggles.
- Encouragers: Downplay the negative effects of the addiction or glorify its perceived benefits.
- Saboteurs: Actively create conditions for relapse, undermining healing efforts.

Enabling often stems from the enabler's own fears and insecurities, such as a fear of losing their own habits, conflict avoidance, fear of rejection, or losing control or purpose if the person recovers.

Enabling behaviours are harmful as they perpetuate the addiction and create unhealthy dynamics of control, limiting the chances of wellbeing for both parties involved.

The Role of Rehab

"One of the hardest things was learning that I was worth recovery." ~ Demi Lovato

Withdrawal from substances or addictive behaviours is not only challenging but can be dangerous, both physically and mentally. This is why medically supervised withdrawal, often provided in inpatient rehabilitation facilities, is essential. Rehab centres, usually located within or near hospitals, provide a structured, safe environment where detox and early recovery can occur with professional oversight.

What Happens in Rehab?

Every rehab facility may manage its programs and its people differently. However, from my experience here are some things that you can expect to see behind closed doors.

Tight security. Entrance and exits may be monitored and even restricted, with manual release of the doors by staff often required. There will be security cameras in public spaces and even a security guard or two around to deal with any major disruptions.

A hospital environment. While some rehabs are made to feel like hotels or resorts, others are more like medical facilities.

As such, the rooms may be fitted with equipment required for medical emergencies, and will have a sterile hospital smell. The rooms will also be devoid of anything that could be used for self-harm, for example, hooks or hangers.

Communal entertainment and meals. People are there to rest and so don't want other residents providing disturbance. For this reason, televisions may only be provided in the common rooms and meals are expected to be taken in the communal dining room.

Bag checks. On check in, and after return from any excursions, it is likely that all bags will be searched for anything that could relate to substance abuse or self-harm.

Medication supervision. Medicine is usually only provided with the doctor's approval and administered by the nursing staff. In all cases, the rehab would use its medication rather than yours, just in case you have found a sneaky way to smuggle contraband into the pills!

Monitoring meals. Nurses may check that you are taking in regular meals, even making notes on your chart to show that you are getting sufficient sustenance.

Restricted movement. In the beginning a person may not be allowed out of the facility, so that they are kept in a safe place while they detox and are put at less risk of relapse. As the healing progresses a resident may be provided with time out, however with strict return times enforced and police intervention possible if they do not come back when required.

Meetings with the medical team. Days are spent working with a number of medical specialists, including the following:

- Psychiatrist – to deal with the cognitive imbalances occurring due to the addiction and work on a medication plan.
- Counsellor – to assist with the mental and emotional patterns that may have led to or are keeping you stuck in addiction.
- General practitioner – to do specific physical checks to determine the extent of damage done through addiction.
- Dietician – to advise how you can restore your body's nutrition and energy levels.
- Nurse – to check your physical and mental welfare during your stay.

Medical examinations and tests. Blood tests and scans of the body and brain are usually conducted to determine how much damage had been done and plan the medical path forward.

Group classes. Structured classes are often provided to assist with a holistic understanding of addiction and to introduce some life skills to begin the process of healing.

Restrictions on visitors. Visitors may not be permitted for the first few days as a detox is undertaken. From then on, any visits may be monitored by staff, and guests to the facility will be required to have their bags checked to ensure they are not bringing in any harmful substances.

Does this description of rehab sound like a prison? Well, in a way, it is. At the very least, it was a severe case of micro-management. There are two schools of thought as to why the initial strict and restrained environment is required to facilitate healing:

- People with an addiction cannot be trusted to manage themselves. The depth of damage to the decision-making functions of the brain means there is some merit to this argument. The patients will find it difficult to make good choices about their care, so these must be made for them until there is some obvious ability to be accountable.

- It frees the patient to concentrate on their healing. When there are fewer choices about where you will go, what you will do and how, this mental energy can be invested into the educational and healing program.

I know many people who struggled with the loss of control when they first entered rehab and found the decreased autonomy, making them anxious and angry. However, this is part of the process of letting go of the person who ended up in this place, but also an integral part of learning how to receive help.

Does Rehab Work?

Well, this is the ultimate question. The answer for each person will be different because it depends on the quality of the rehab facility and the mindset of the person entering it. I am willing to admit that rehab certainly didn't work for me…. the first four times. Yep, that's right; I was the one making jokes about getting a frequent flyer card and asking how many admissions you have to buy before I would get one free. However, all these jokes were only masking the deep shame and despair of a relapse. Humour was the way I coped with once again being a 'patient', losing autonomy and what I considered freedom.

And then came admission number five.

What was the difference with admission number five?

A Proactive Admission

My fifth visit to rehab was my first proactive admission. By proactive, I mean that I requested to be admitted rather than going through a relapse, being made go in for detox and forced to stay to get back on track. My medical team was always saying I was welcome to come back anytime. I should not wait to be struggling desperately to get some help. So, with the help from my psych, I identified the most vulnerable time for me to relapse during the school holidays. Holidays were when routines went out the window. I was exhausted from the school term and had the chance to spend some time alone. These factors presented both the desire to seek comfort in my substance and the opportunity to do so. So, my fifth admission to rehab was proactively scheduled for the next school holidays.

Walking into rehab for the first time sober and not in the throes of withdrawal was so empowering. I felt strong, felt in control of my destiny, and knew I had turned a corner in my healing. I knew that I was finally learning what rehab is there to do – teach you to care for yourself. So why didn't the first six times work? On reflection, I can see three key reasons:

Faulty Expectations

I am sure my family and I were not alone in thinking that I would walk out of my first stint in rehab 'cured.' My doctor did counsel me that this was unlikely. Still, I was so desperate for a miracle I went in believing that this one visit to rehab would be the solution to my addiction. So, my definition of what it meant for rehab to work was delivering an all-out magical cure. It was only when I left the first time and began to experience life at home without a crutch did I realised how misguided I was.

When I left rehab the first time, I never could have understood how cruel the cravings would be. I wouldn't have thought I would begin reminiscing about a substance that almost killed me. And I never could have imagined that I would consider throwing away those weeks of isolation and separation from my family by drinking again. But I did.

By going into rehab with these unrealistic expectations, everyone got hurt. My family was bitterly disappointed when I had to return, and I certainly felt like a failure. Looking back, I wish they had a big sign in every room of rehab saying:

"This rehab is not a cure.

It is a step in your journey of healing.

The number of steps it takes to heal differs for every person.

We are here to support you until you can walk these steps on your own."

Maybe if I had read this each day, I would have understood that this first visit, the second visit, and every visit from then on was part of my healing journey and not, as I saw it, marks on a loser's scoreboard.

Lack of Commitment

I will admit that during the first few admissions, I told everyone I was committed to abstinence. In all honesty, I was only committed to figuring out how I could get away with drinking. I remember sitting in the classes scheming about how I could fiddle with my medication and negotiate a drink or two on the holidays. All the while, though, there was an ache in my heart. The ache was a sign I knew I was not honest with myself and was selling myself short. It was a clear signal that I knew I was disrespecting the time of my medical team and family.

And yet, that was the stage of the journey I was at. As you may have read in my article Why Don't I Feel Any Better – the brain and the body take time to heal. You can't just wave a magic wand and repair the wounds caused and the habits formed from years of abuse. My brain was still healing, but I did not recognise or respect how much time it would take. While it was true that I was not fully committed to the process, this did come eventually. But it only came after the brain and body were back to normal functioning.

The analogy I use is a person recovering from a knee replacement. As much as they might desperately want to run a marathon, they can't right now. They can, though, in the future if they support their body to heal, nurture and care for themselves, and begin a sensible training regime. I see it the same way for a person suffering from addiction. Yes, they desperately want to stop being addicted, but first, they need to find support and allow themselves to heal. Rehab is where you get the support for this healing and begin your training for the adventure that is your life.

Needing Someone to Care

I find this to be the saddest reason of all for my repeated return to rehab. When I realised it, though, it was a luminescent lightbulb moment. You see, in rehab, I felt cared for. People were paying me attention. Even if it was just the daily observation and medication sessions, I had people checking on me and asking how I felt. The psychs and counsellors listened, were empathetic and were helping me understand myself. The cooks were concerned with me getting well-fed and healthy again. Even the night checks with torchlight were a great comfort, knowing that someone was looking out for me.

This care was far from the bitterness, anger, lack of trust and apathy that permeated my close relationships. At one stage, I had no friends left, and my partner had completely given up. Any lapse would result in some form of drawn-out psychological punishment. I don't blame anyone. My behaviour was disgusting. But I was desperate for someone to care for me. While I lay silently in my bed, my heart was screaming out for someone to wrap me up, hold me and let me know it would all be ok. While I didn't get this at rehab, it was sure a hell of a lot closer than the outright ostracism I received at home.

If I did develop a reliance upon rehab, it soon came with understanding the gaps I was looking to fill by being there. Every visit, I learnt something new about myself and the healing journey. Each discussion with other residents, nurses, or doctors helped me become stronger to start giving this same care to myself. While yes, in some ways, rehab had become a retreat, it was also the place where I got to practice the most basic forms of self-care that strengthened the foundation for my next step.

The Role of Rehab

So, yes, in the beginning, I thought that rehab was not working. Everyone around me agreed. In hindsight, though, rehab was working because it has:

- Provided me with a safe place to detox.
- Helped me understand the journey of healing.
- Provided much-needed care and support for the healing process.
- Given me an effective training ground to learn how to care for myself.

And this seems to be the true role of rehab. People with addictions have hated and harmed themselves for a long time. In fact, for some, they may never have known what it is like to know, respect and love themselves fully. Rehab is not a magic wand that can make these years of trauma disappear. It is there to help people through the long and difficult healing journey, but more importantly, to help them learn how to love and care for themselves. This is the greatest gift.

You can't put a number on the number of visits to rehab that learning to love yourself will take. I would say there is no 'finish line' to self-love. It is a practice and a life-long dedication. But I know that when you are willing to be honest with yourself about where you are, you have taken huge leaps ahead. Until such time, reach out to all the support that is available for you. Every day is another step on your journey, and when you get support, you become stronger and more able to take the next step on your own.

What If I Can't Get Into Rehab?

This question is real for so many people. People need help, and to think that they can't get it because of financial status, the fine print on insurance plans, or lack of capacity is heartbreaking. But this does not mean you just give up. While in rehab, you have access to all types of medical assistance in one place. However, there is nothing to say that you can't create your own team right where you are.

The first place to start is by finding a good general practitioner. These are priceless, and please treat them like the precious gems that they are. A great doctor will support you through withdrawal or refer you to an outpatient clinic that can provide you with what you need to do it safely. The doctor will do the tests necessary to identify any physical damage done during the addiction and refer you to psychiatrists, counsellors, and dieticians to deal with the other physical and emotional trauma. While they can't do everything for you, a good doctor will find the people who can.

Building your own rehab team will certainly take a more invested effort on your behalf. It is a great idea to do your own research before meeting with your doctor about services or professionals in the area you would like to be referred to, making your doctor's task a lot easier. Ultimately, you will need to take over the reins of your healing. So, in a way, this approach of setting up your own rehab team is just bringing this responsibility forward.

Core Concepts

Rehab provides medical support during withdrawal in a controlled, often hospital-like environment.

Facilities are designed for safety, with strict protocols like bag checks and monitored interactions, to minimise risks of substance abuse or self-harm.

Patients engage with a team of medical professionals, including psychiatrists, counsellors, dietitians, and general practitioners, to address the cognitive, emotional, and physical aspects of addiction.

Some may enter rehab expecting an immediate cure, but it's a step in a longer journey of healing.

Rehabilitation is a training ground for self-care, helping individuals learn how to respect and nurture themselves.

Repeated admissions are not failures but opportunities to learn about personal triggers, needs, and the importance of proactive engagement in recovery.

A proactive approach, such as entering rehab before a relapse, can be empowering and transformative.

For those unable to access rehab, building a personal support team with a good general practitioner is crucial.

Section 7- Key Challenges in Healing from Addiction

The Cruelty of Cravings

Navigating cravings, one at a time, with self-compassion and resilience, is an act of immense courage.

Cravings are often among the most challenging withdrawal symptoms, representing an intense pull or overwhelming desire to return to the addictive substance or behaviour. These cravings can be relentless, feeling like taunting spectres that lure individuals back into self-harm just when they have committed to breaking free. The experience of cravings can be profoundly disheartening, especially when the mind begins to scheme ways to abandon detox and return to addiction. In these moments, the depth of one's internal struggle is fully revealed, as well as the remarkable, albeit misdirected, resourcefulness and persistence of the addicted mind. If only this energy and passion could be channelled into more constructive pursuits.

Cravings should not merely be seen as tests of commitment but as opportunities to learn self-care and self-love. They are not just distressing and challenging, but also a chance to develop invaluable skills for overcoming life's obstacles.

Understanding the Nature of Cravings

From my experience I feel that there are two distinct kinds of cravings:

1. Cravings that are like a crisis - overwhelming waves that feel like an emergency.

2. Cravings that feel like chronic pain - troubling emotions that hang heavily and persistently in the back of your mind.

During the early stages of detox and healing, cravings often present as the first type, an intense and urgent, necessitating an immediate and focused response. Over time, as the healing process progresses, these may dull in intensity, but not always immediately in frequency. It can take many months for a person to be able to separate themselves from the urges and create space between the craving and the response.

The Emergency Response to Cravings

When cravings feel like an emergency—when they are too intense and overwhelming to manage calmly—it is important to approach them as one would any other crisis. The essential skill of crisis management found later in this book is applicable to cravings. Early in the healing process, cravings are a common form of emotional crisis, and treating them with appropriate care and compassion can help prevent acting on these intense urges.

Extreme cravings often trap individuals in a cognitive and emotional loop, as illustrated in the following diagram. This cycle typically unfolds as follows:

- A sensation of craving arises.
- Feelings of guilt or shame emerge in response to the craving.
- Self-doubt begins to creep in, questioning the ability to change.

- Further guilt and shame develop from the perception of being a failure.
- Efforts to avoid these painful emotions intensify.
- The craving for the substance or activity strengthens to dull the hurt.

Figure 15 - The Downward Spiral of a Craving

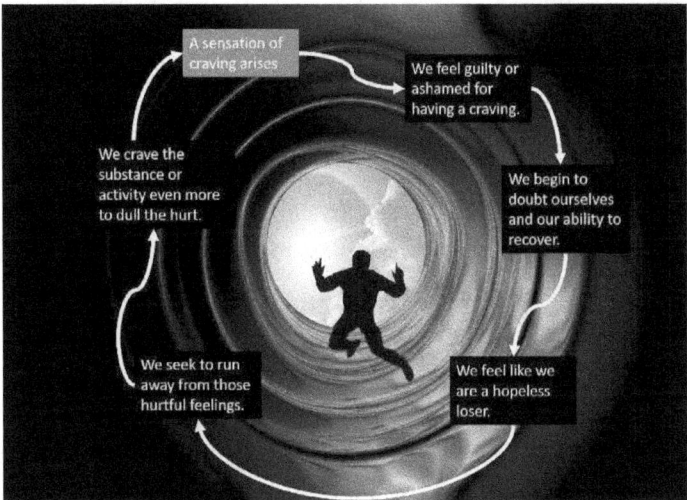

Breaking this cycle requires intervention to disrupt the pattern of self-defeating thoughts and painful emotions. While in the past, extreme measures like a slap in the face were sometimes used to break hysteria, modern approaches focus on grounding techniques that bring awareness back to the present moment. This interruption is crucial in halting the downward spiral. Learning and applying crisis management skills is empowering and essential, as it enables individuals to recognise when they have entered crisis mode and provides them with tools to regain equilibrium.

Treating Cravings Like Difficult Emotions

It is true; cravings hold great suffering. They are born from a past of repeated self-harm. And they are the traumatic reality of the present. But they are not your future. They will dwindle, and they will someday cease. But in the meantime, you can use them to build strength to deal with the many other difficult emotions that will come your way. In the past, you have used your substance or activity to run away from these emotions. Now is the time to get brave. Now is the time to create the foundation for true healing.

The fact is, if you want to heal from an addiction fully, you are going to have to learn how to deal with difficult emotions. Cravings are just one of the feelings that are here right now for you to learn from. It is not pretty, it is not pleasant, but if you are willing to brave, the process of sitting with, and caring for your cravings is completely empowering. And the reality is, dealing with difficult emotions does take courage. It is easier to push them away, to suppress them, but know they will fester and come back bigger and more destructive. The only way to deal with difficult emotions is to care for them.

Pema Chodron calls this 'leaning into the discomfort. In her book *Taking the Leap: Freeing Ourselves from Old Habits and Fears*, she says:

"The next time you lose heart, and you can't bear to experience what you're feeling, you might recall this instruction: change the way you see it and lean in. Instead of blaming our discomfort on outer circumstances or our

weakness, we can choose to stay present and awake to our experience. Not rejecting it, not grasping it, not buying the stories that we relentlessly tell ourselves. This is priceless advice that addresses the true cause of suffering - yours, mine, and that of all living beings." ~ Pema Chodron

Pema tells us that instead of trying to push our cravings away, and use them to reinforce our feelings of failure, we have the chance to care for them, to be present with the experience and lean into the pain. For leaning into the discomfort is a practice of courage and compassion.

Seeking Support

Managing cravings can be an isolating experience, but it is important to remember that seeking support is not a sign of weakness; rather, it is a demonstration of genuine strength and courage. You are not alone in this journey. Many individuals and support systems are available, eager to assist in navigating these challenging moments. The bravery required to confront and manage cravings should not be underestimated. As poignantly illustrated in the quote from Charlie Mackesy's *The Boy, the Mole, the Fox and the Horse*:

"'What's the bravest thing you've ever said?' asked the boy.

'Help,' said the horse."

Cravings represent a difficult but integral part of the healing journey, offering both challenge and opportunity. By responding with self-compassion, reaching out for support, and employing crisis management tools, the grip of cravings can be loosened, making way for continued progress on the path to healing.

Core Concepts

Cravings are one of the most challenging aspects of withdrawal, presenting as intense urges to return to addictive behaviours. They often feel overwhelming and can lead to a cycle of self-doubt, guilt, and shame.

Navigating cravings with resilience and self-compassion is crucial, as they offer opportunities to develop skills in self-care and self-love.

Cravings can range from overwhelming, urgent sensations to persistent but subtle thoughts.

Early in healing, cravings often feel like crises, requiring immediate grounding techniques to break the cycle of negative emotions and prevent relapse.

Treat extreme cravings like an emotional crisis and use crisis management skills to disrupt harmful patterns.

Seeking support and asking for help is an act of courage, not weakness, and can be instrumental in managing cravings effectively.

The Nasty Side Effect of Anhedonia

"Sometimes, carrying on, just carrying on, is the superhuman achievement." ~ *Albert Camus*

Anhedonia, a condition that is more common than you might think, is often experienced during the healing process from addiction. It's marked by an inability to feel pleasure in everyday activities, creating a state of emotional numbness that can be disheartening. This sense of emptiness and disconnection from life's joys is a challenging part of the healing journey for many, and poses a significant risk for relapse due to the discouragement it can bring.

I know this discouragement intimately. After months of following the recommended steps of healing—eating well, taking medication, exercising, socialising, and maintaining a regular sleep schedule—I still felt like I was walking through a fog. I was constantly plagued by an overwhelming sense of blankness. There was no enjoyment of simple pleasures, like the taste of fresh strawberries at breakfast, the warmth of the sun during a beach walk, or the emotions stirred by a book. Even after a good night's sleep, there was no sense of refreshment or revitalisation. Social interactions felt hollow, with an underlying awareness that participation was merely a surface-level act, disconnected from any genuine emotional engagement.

This state persisted for six months, during which the absence of feeling and the growing sadness led to the thought that perhaps it was this void that had driven the initial turn to alcohol. The despair eventually led to a relapse, and after just two weeks, there was a return to rehab, accompanied by a crushing sense of failure. It was only through discussions with counsellors that the condition was identified as Anhedonia, a term that captures this inability to feel pleasure in normal activities.

Anhedonia is common in the initial months of withdrawal and can extend up to two years. It may be linked to medications used for treating depression and withdrawal symptoms, or it may simply be a part of the natural healing process. Studies indicate that Anhedonia is associated with an increase in cravings and a higher likelihood of relapse. Therefore, it is crucial to have realistic expectations about the time it takes for emotional responses to return. Understanding that it might take a year or more for feelings to resurface can foster a gentler and more patient approach to oneself during healing.

During the recovery process, it's crucial to remember that the brain's pleasure centres, like any other part of the body, require time to recover from the intense assault of artificial stimuli that addiction often involves. This is a period where patience and self-compassion are essential. The advice often given is to 'act as if' or 'fake it 'til you make it,' which can feel frustrating or even dismissive at first. For someone in the grips of Anhedonia, these suggestions can seem out of touch with the depth of despair felt, as it might seem impossible to merely 'act' happy or engaged when the inner reality is one of profound disconnection.

It's important to understand that healing the brain's pleasure centres is a gradual process, and there is no set timeframe. The return of pleasure is not immediate, and it's not something that can be forced. The only approach is to continue with actions aligning with one's values and desired outcomes, even when those actions do not bring joy. Over time, this persistence can restore trust between the self and the brain, demonstrating that the body and mind are no longer being subjected to the harmful substances or activities that caused the damage.

Escaping from Anhedonia is not just a possibility, it's a reality. The sensations do return. For some, it may take well over a year, but one day, the small joys of life begin to reappear—like the taste of a strawberry or the rush of endorphins from exercise. Each small return of feeling serves as a powerful reminder of the progress made and the resilience built along the way.

This process of regaining pleasure in life requires trust, patience, and a commitment to self-care. The brain's pleasure centre, which retreats into a protective mode during periods of severe distress, needs time to heal and to relearn the enjoyment that come with a healthier life. As this trust is rebuilt, the natural flow of pleasurable feelings will begin to return, marking a significant milestone in the journey of healing.

Core Concepts

Anhedonia, or the inability to feel pleasure, is common during the initial months of withdrawal and can persist for up to two years. It results in a sense of emotional numbness and disconnection, posing a significant risk for relapse.

This condition may stem from medication side effects or as part of the natural healing process. It is crucial to have realistic expectations about the time it takes for emotional responses to return.

Anhedonia can make daily activities feel meaningless, leading to thoughts of relapse due to the lack of emotional engagement or joy.

Understanding that pleasure will eventually return can help foster patience and self-compassion during the healing process. Acting in alignment with values, even without immediate joy, supports the gradual restoration of the brain's pleasure centres.

Healing from anhedonia requires trust, persistence, and self-care. As the brain recovers, small joys gradually re-emerge, marking progress and reinforcing resilience.

The journey back to experiencing pleasure is slow but achievable, with each small return of feeling serving as a reminder of the body and mind's capacity to heal and thrive.

The Reality of Relapse

"You may encounter many defeats, but you must not be defeated. It may be necessary to encounter the defeats, so you can know who you are, what you can rise from, how you can still come out of it." — Maya Angelou.

While the journey through healing from addiction may be envisioned as smooth and straightforward, the reality often involves encountering significant obstacles. These challenges can range from minor setbacks that are easy to overcome to more severe relapses that can feel overwhelming. However, three truths remain constant:

1. Challenges are inevitable.
2. They offer opportunities for growth.
3. They will pass.

Obstacles arise because healing involves change - either engaging in new activities or altering the way you do existing ones. Without these challenges, the potential for personal growth and self-discovery would be limited. Each success and setback on this journey hold valuable lessons that contribute to a deeper understanding of oneself and one's strengths. As the saying goes, a great sailor is forged through navigating rough seas, just as a resilient life is built upon overcoming failures.

"It's fine to celebrate success, but it is more important to heed the lessons of failure." — Bill Gates.

Amid a challenging situation, seeing beyond the immediate discomfort may be difficult. However, recognising that such moments are transient can help shift the focus to how best to respond. While external circumstances may be beyond control, the choice of response remains a powerful tool. Rather than succumbing to panic or negative thought cycles, grounding oneself in calm and compassionate actions can nurture resilience.

Understanding Relapse

Relapse is one of the most disheartening setbacks in the healing process. A period of sobriety often brings restored confidence and renewed hope, which can make a relapse feel like a devastating blow. This experience can be compounded by the reactions of others, who may express doubt or criticism, amplifying feelings of failure. The key is to act swiftly and focus on the steps needed to regain stability rather than dwelling on the relapse itself, which is now in the past and cannot be changed.

Initial Steps to Take After a Relapse

1. Breathe

The first and most crucial step is to breathe. This simple action can help calm the body's stress response, which is often triggered during moments of anxiety or distress. Deep breathing activates the parasympathetic nervous system, allowing the mind to regain clarity and composure. If breathing alone does not sufficiently manage the emotional response, further crisis management techniques, such as those provided later in this book, may be necessary.

As you work through the relapse, re-establishing the other elements of Base Camp - nutrition, movement, sleep and medication - will also be important.

2. Get Real

Facing the reality of the situation is the next essential step. Acknowledging the following facts can help in processing the relapse:

You are unwinding automatic behaviours: Addictive behaviours are deeply embedded in the brain's neural pathways, and changing these patterns takes time. Understanding that these behaviours are automatic and will resurface is part of the process, not an excuse but a context for self-compassion.

The journey is a learning process: healing is about learning—learning about addiction, oneself, and new ways of living. Viewing relapses as part of the learning curve rather than failures can shift the focus toward growth. Just as children are not reprimanded for stumbling while learning to walk, self-compassion is essential during moments of struggle.

Healing is a cumulative process, not a restart. A common misconception is that relapse resets progress to zero. In reality, every day of sobriety contributes to the overall journey. Recognising and celebrating periods of sobriety, no matter their length, reinforces that each moment contributes to healing. A relapse does not erase progress; it adds to the cumulative learning and growth experience.

Others' reactions may exacerbate feelings of failure: The responses of others can intensify the emotional impact of a relapse. While it is natural to feel affected by criticism or disappointment from others, maintaining a focus on personal actions and responses is crucial. Distancing oneself emotionally from negative reactions and concentrating on the next steps is a constructive approach.

Moving Forward: The CARE Approach

After grounding in reality, the next phase involves taking deliberate actions to move forward. The CARE approach outlines four steps to help regain momentum:

C - Call someone

Reach out for support immediately. Whether it is a trusted friend, a counsellor, a helpline, or an online support group, connecting with others can provide the necessary accountability and encouragement to start moving forward again. Isolation can lead to overthinking and self-judgment, making it essential to seek connection rather than retreat.

A - Acknowledge the situation

Recognise and validate the emotional response to the relapse. Acknowledging feelings of disappointment, shame, or frustration is an act of self-compassion. Suppressing or denying these emotions may prolong distress, whereas accepting them can facilitate healing. Emotions, like waves, will eventually pass when allowed to flow naturally.

R - Release guilt

Guilt and shame are powerful emotions that can hinder progress. While these feelings may signal a commitment to healing, clinging to them can keep one stuck. Acknowledging regret for the relapse is a healthier alternative, as it allows for reflection and the motivation to take corrective action without being immobilised by negative emotions.

E - Educate and reflect

Relapse offers an opportunity to learn and adjust strategies for healing. Reflecting on the experience with honesty can reveal critical insights. Consider asking the following questions, either alone or with a support network:

- What strategies were effective before the relapse?
- What areas were challenging or less effective?
- How well did I maintain my Base Camp?
- Were there specific triggers, such as people, environments, thoughts, or emotions, which contributed to the relapse?
- Were there moments where a different choice could have been made?
- What actions will be continued, and what new strategies can be implemented moving forward?

Regular review and reflection are invaluable practices throughout the healing journey. By consistently assessing what works and what does not, the approach to healing can be continually refined. The power to create change lies within, and a commitment to learning from each experience is key to that empowerment.

By taking proactive steps, even after setbacks, the journey towards healing remains on course. Relapse does not define the individual but serves as a stepping stone toward greater resilience and understanding. Each challenge, when met with care and self-compassion, becomes an integral part of the transformative process of healing.

Core Concepts

Relapse is a return to addictive behaviours after a period of sobriety.

Relapses are only failures if there is no learning from them. Each relapse presents a chance to learn and refine one's approach to healing.

Healing is cumulative; a relapse does not erase progress made previously.

The key is to respond quickly, focus on regaining stability, and avoid dwelling on the past.

Initial Steps After Relapse:
- Breathe: Start by calming your body and mind with deep breathing to regain composure.
- Get Real: Acknowledge the reality of relapse by understanding:
  - Addictive behaviours are deeply ingrained and take time to change.
  - The reactions of others can enflame negative reactions or derail positive ones. Choose helpers here wisely.

Moving Forward: The CARE Approach:
- C - Call someone: Reach out for support from friends, counsellors, or support groups.
- A - Acknowledge the situation: Validate your feelings of disappointment or frustration.
- R - Release guilt: Let go of guilt and shame, which can hinder progress.
- E - Educate and reflect: Use the relapse as a learning opportunity. Adjust strategies to better handle future challenges.

Rebuilding Trust

"Trust is not won by words, but by actions." ~ Anonymous

Trust—defined as the firm belief in the reliability, truth, or ability of someone or something—is often a significant casualty in the context of addiction. Addiction creates a relentless pursuit of substances or activities that the brain mistakenly equates with survival. This pursuit often results in the neglect of health, career, and relationships. The impact on personal connections is severe, as addiction can lead to lies, deceit, and manipulation, and an inability to fulfil commitments.

The Erosion of Trust in Relationships

Trust is the foundation of any relationship, acting as a stabilising force that enables connection and mutual support. In the throes of addiction, individuals may become unreliable, unable to maintain sobriety or effectively undertake their basic responsibilities. Repeated relapses can further erode others' confidence in the individual's level of care for their loved ones, and ability to overcome addiction. When trust is compromised, relationships weaken, leaving individuals isolated and disconnected at a time when they most need support.

However, the presence of addiction can create a toxic environment for those around the individual, breeding fear, anxiety, and a sense of instability. In such circumstances, it is crucial for family members, friends, and colleagues to protect their own wellbeing, which may sometimes involve setting boundaries or distancing themselves from the person struggling with addiction.

The Loss of Self-Trust

Arguably, one of the most profound consequences of addiction is the loss of self-trust. Doubting oneself can undermine the foundation necessary for recovery. This loss often manifests as a lack of faith in one's ability to make sound decisions, be truthful, or sustain efforts to overcome addiction. Self-trust is critical for genuine healing, as it involves a commitment to authenticity and self-care across physical, mental, and spiritual dimensions.

Rebuilding Self-Trust: A Pathway to Healing

Rebuilding self-trust is not an easy task; it requires consistent effort and dedication. Self-trust is not simply restored through affirmations or external validation—it is earned through repeated actions that align with one's values and commitments. This process begins with honesty, particularly self-honesty, which forms the cornerstone of trust.

The path to restoring self-trust starts with acknowledging the truth of one's experiences and vulnerabilities. This honesty must first be directed inward, as the facade of perfection often masks deeper fears of acceptance and self-worth. Genuine self-acceptance is a crucial step in reconnecting with one's authentic self and nurturing the healing process.

The Role of Consistent Action in Rebuilding Trust

Rebuilding self-trust in the wake of addiction is a gradual process that hinges on consistent action. Trust is not restored overnight; it is cultivated through a series of small, deliberate steps that reinforce a commitment to oneself. The key to this process lies in following through on even the tiniest commitments, which collectively build a foundation of reliability and self-respect.

The Power of Small, Frequent Steps

The path to reestablishing self-trust often begins with minor, manageable actions. These can be as simple as committing to a daily routine, such as waking up at a certain time, practicing self-care, or keeping promises made to oneself, like attending a support group or engaging in a brief exercise routine. Each small action, when completed consistently, serves as evidence that the individual can make decisions and sticking to them. This incremental approach makes the daunting task of rebuilding trust more approachable and sustainable.

Each step, no matter how small, contributes to a growing sense of self-efficacy—the belief in one's ability to succeed. This belief is critical in the recovery journey, as it counters the pervasive self-doubt that often accompanies addiction. As individuals demonstrate to themselves that they can follow through on small commitments, they begin to challenge the narrative that they are unreliable or incapable of change. Over time, these small victories accumulate, creating a positive feedback loop that reinforces self-trust.

Following Through on Commitments

The act of following through on commitments, even the most minor ones, is a powerful testament to one's integrity and reliability. For someone recovering from addiction, where broken promises and failed attempts may have been a common experience, the importance of following through cannot be overstated. Each fulfilled commitment is a step towards mending the internal rift caused by past actions and begins to rebuild the foundation of self-trust.

This consistency in action demonstrates to the individual that they are capable of making choices that align with their values and long-term goals. Whether it's staying sober for another day, choosing healthier foods, or simply showing up on time, each fulfilled commitment sends a clear message: "I am someone who can be trusted to do what I say I will do." This message is crucial for restoring a positive self-image and overcoming the self-doubt that often lingers from past behaviours associated with addiction.

The Cumulative Effect of Consistency

Consistency is the cornerstone of rebuilding trust. The cumulative effect of small, consistent actions is far greater than any single grand gesture. It's the daily choices and actions that quietly, yet powerfully, restore confidence in one's ability to manage life and its challenges. Over time, these actions foster a sense of stability and predictability, not only for oneself but also in relationships with others.

This approach also helps in managing setbacks, such as relapses, which can otherwise feel overwhelming. By focusing on maintaining consistency in small actions, individuals can quickly regain their footing after a stumble, rather than feeling as though they are starting over from scratch. This resilience further strengthens self-trust, as it affirms the individual's capacity to navigate difficulties without losing sight of their broader healing journey.

Building a Foundation of Reliability

Reliability is the bedrock of trust. By prioritizing consistent, small steps, individuals in recovery can gradually rebuild their reliability, both in their own eyes and in the eyes of others. This process requires patience and self-compassion, recognizing that trust is not rebuilt through perfection, but through persistence and honesty. Each day offers a new opportunity to take actions that honour one's commitments and values, contributing to a stronger, more resilient foundation of self-trust.

Ultimately, the journey to reestablish trust is about showing up for oneself, time and time again. It's about proving, through action, that one is committed to the path of healing, not just in words, but in deeds. This steady, deliberate approach to rebuilding trust creates a powerful momentum that carries individuals forward, guiding them toward a future defined by integrity, self-respect, and a renewed connection with their true selves.

It May Take Others Longer to Trust Again

It is important to acknowledge that rebuilding trust with others may take longer. While the individual may feel a renewed sense of direction and purpose, those around them may still carry the scars of past betrayals and disappointments. They will not easily forget how much pain and trouble has been caused and to protect themselves from further heartache, may hold back from trusting until they can be confident that changes not only have been made but are cemented. Reestablishing trust with loved ones requires patience and consistent demonstrations of reliability and integrity.

Moving Forward with Self-Trust

The most crucial relationship to mend is the one with oneself. Trust in one's own spirit provides the strength and guidance needed to navigate the complexities of addiction and recovery. By committing to actions that reflect integrity and care, individuals can begin to heal not only themselves but also the relationships that were damaged along the way. Rebuilding self-trust fosters resilience and offers a pathway to a life of authenticity, connection, and fulfillment.

Core Concepts

Trust is often lost during addiction, leading to unreliability, deceit, and damaged relationships. This loss also extends to self-trust, creating doubt in one's ability to make sound decisions.

Rebuilding self-trust requires consistent, honest actions and self-acceptance, demonstrating integrity through repeated small steps that align with personal values.

Small, manageable actions—like keeping promises and maintaining routines—help restore self-efficacy, proving to oneself that change is possible.

The cumulative effect of small, consistent actions is powerful, fostering stability and providing a means to handle setbacks like relapses without feeling as though all progress is lost.

Rebuilding trust with others takes time, as they may still carry the hurt from past betrayals.

The most important relationship to repair, however, is with oneself. By committing to actions that reflect care and honesty, individuals can rebuild self-trust.

Sending Care to the Carers

"The simple act of caring is heroic." ~ *Edward Albert*

Caring for someone with an addiction is an emotionally taxing experience that often brings feelings of helplessness and uncertainty. The journey of supporting a loved one through addiction is complex and fraught with challenges. It is natural to have questions like, "When will this end?" or "Do I have the strength to endure this?" While these questions cannot be easily answered, sharing experiences from those who have navigated the path of healing may offer some insights and support.

For individuals struggling with addiction, the journey toward healing is not only a physical endeavour but also one that requires deep emotional and spiritual work. It often involves confronting and shedding layers of shame and guilt to live a more fulfilling life. The process is typically long, difficult, and sometimes traumatic. As someone who has personally progressed through this journey, it has taken several years to regain confidence and a sense of stability. Recognising the depth and complexity of the healing process can be essential for both the individual in healing and their carers.

Those who care for individuals with addiction also experience a parallel healing journey filled with its own set of challenges and traumas. Carers often endure significant emotional stress, experience shame and guilt, and navigate the tumultuous ups and downs of their loved one's healing journey. They are also likely to battle with thoughts about how they may have contributed to the chaos, and how they too may need to change to improve their own wellbeing.

Common Challenges Faced by Carers

Carers may struggle with several issues, including a lack of control, coping with relapses, and caregiver fatigue. Understanding these challenges and exploring strategies to manage them can help maintain the carer's wellbeing and capacity to support their loved one.

1. Lack of Control

One of the most immediate and difficult realisations in caring for someone with addiction is the lack of control over the situation. Addiction fundamentally alters brain function, often prioritizing the addictive substance or behaviour above all else. This shift can make it seem like the individual is no longer fully in control of their decisions. Similarly, carers may feel powerless in influencing their loved one's behaviour.

Carers may find themselves in a constant state of worry, trying to determine the best course of action. However, it is important to acknowledge that the only actions within one's control are one's own. Expending energy on attempts to control the behaviour of a loved one can be draining and unproductive. Instead, carers are encouraged to focus on what they can influence. A practical tool for navigating these situations is the Decision-Making Matrix, a tool that helps individuals assess an issue's importance and their ability to control or influence it. By using this tool, carers can make more informed and balanced decisions in the face of complex and emotionally charged situations.

Figure 16 - The Decision-Making Matrix for Carers

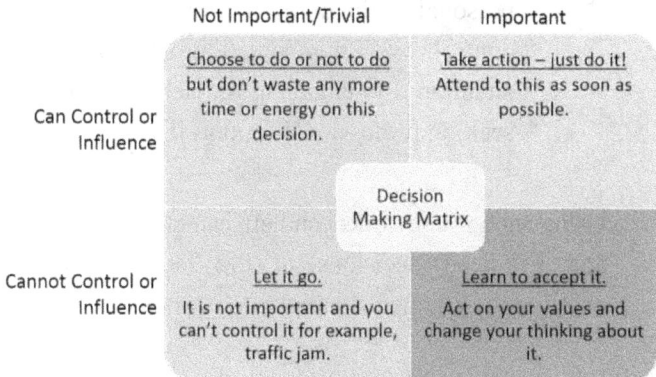

	Not Important/Trivial	Important
Can Control or Influence	Choose to do or not to do but don't waste any more time or energy on this decision.	Take action – just do it! Attend to this as soon as possible.
		Decision Making Matrix
Cannot Control or Influence	Let it go. It is not important and you can't control it for example, traffic jam.	Learn to accept it. Act on your values and change your thinking about it.

Here are some examples of how the Decision-Making Matrix can be used to regain a sense of perspective over common carer issues:

- If a loved one is not seeking help for their addiction, then this is definitely an important issue as it affects their health and relationships. And there is something the carer can do about it. They can seek guidance from professionals and consult with healthcare providers about the options available to help their loved one.

- If a recently rehabilitated individual has one glass of wine at dinner, then while it may feel like a huge failure, in the scheme of their full recover it is minor. The carer cannot control this situation as the person is an adult and has autonomy. Instead, the carer may need to let this one go without making it an area of focus and choose to communicate calmly after the dinner.

- Feeling overwhelmed by the caregiving role is definitely an important issue because maintaining personal wellbeing is critical. A caregiver does have control over this situation and can address the situation by engaging in self-care activities and seeking professional support if needed.

Using such frameworks can help carers make more informed and balanced decisions in the face of complex and emotionally charged situations.

2. Coping with Relapse

Relapses are a common and often distressing aspect of the healing process. They can undermine the progress made during periods of sobriety and reignite doubts and fears for both the individual and their carers. While relapses are challenging, they are not definitive failures. Recognising this can help in managing the emotional impact of a relapse.

In times of relapse, carers are encouraged to take the following steps to manage the situation constructively:

- **Breathe**: Taking time to breathe deeply and engage the parasympathetic nervous system can help calm the body and mind, allowing carers to respond more thoughtfully rather than react impulsively out of fear or frustration.

- **Get Real**: Understanding the nature of addiction as a long-term process with potential setbacks can shift the perspective from seeing relapse as a failure to viewing it as a learning opportunity. This involves acknowledging that addictive behaviours are deeply ingrained and may take time to unlearn and that each period of sobriety, no matter how brief, contributes to overall progress.

- **Moderate Responses**: The reaction of carers can significantly influence the emotional state of the individual in healing. Harsh reactions, such as anger or blame, may deepen feelings of shame and potentially trigger further relapse. Instead, carers are encouraged to respond with understanding and support or, if unable to do so constructively, to step back until they can engage from a place of calm and care.

- **Seeking professional support** is crucial for carers. Reaching out to a support network, whether through friends, professionals, or online communities, can provide the necessary emotional and practical assistance during difficult times. Professional support can offer guidance, coping strategies, and a safe space to express feelings and concerns.

3. Caregiver Fatigue

Caring for someone with addiction can lead to caregiver fatigue, a condition characterized by emotional, mental, and physical exhaustion. Symptoms may include intolerance, resentment, apathy, disengagement, sleep disturbances, and physical ailments such as headaches or nausea. Caregiver fatigue can erode the carer's capacity to provide effective support and compromise their health.

Carers must see these signs early and take proactive steps to address them. Prioritizing self-care is not an act of selfishness but a necessary measure to ensure sustainability in the caregiving role. Engaging in activities that replenish energy, seeking professional support, and setting healthy boundaries are crucial strategies for managing caregiver fatigue. By taking care of themselves, carers can feel empowered and capable of managing their responsibilities.

Caring for a loved one with addiction is undoubtedly a demanding and often overwhelming experience. However, by understanding the limits of one's control, managing responses to setbacks such as relapses, and actively addressing caregiver fatigue, carers can maintain their wellbeing and continue to provide the support their loved ones need. The journey of healing is not just for the individual with addiction but also for those who care for them. Carers can find resilience and hope along this shared path through patience, understanding, and self-care, feeling connected and less isolated in their experiences.

Core Concepts

Caring for someone with addiction is emotionally taxing, often filled with helplessness, uncertainty, and personal challenges.

Carers face their own parallel journey, dealing with emotional stress and uncertainty, shame, guilt and fear.

Common Challenges Faced by Carers:
- Lack of Control: Carers often feel powerless as addiction alters priorities and behaviours. Focusing on what can be controlled helps preserve energy and effectiveness.
- Coping with Relapse: Relapses are common and disheartening but are only failures if there is no learning gained. Carers should manage their response to relapses by:
  - Breathing to stay calm and composed.
  - Acknowledging that setbacks are part of the long-term healing process.
  - Responding with understanding rather than anger or blame to avoid deepening shame.
  - Seeking professional support for guidance and emotional support.
- Caregiver Fatigue: Symptoms include exhaustion, intolerance, disengagement, sleep issues, and physical ailments.

Recognising early signs of carer fatigue and prioritising self-care is essential.

Strategies to address carer fatigue include engaging in energy-replenishing activities, establishing a solid support team for themselves, and setting boundaries.

Section 8- Essential Skills

Essential Skill: Crisis Management

"When written in Chinese, the word crisis is composed of two characters - one represents danger, and the other represents opportunity."

— John F. Kennedy

During the healing journey, there may be moments when emotions feel overwhelming, akin to being caught in a tsunami. Such intense emotional waves can manifest as powerful cravings for a substance or activity, accompanied by a mixture of desire and despair. Additionally, emotions such as guilt and shame related to past actions can be equally overwhelming, potentially leading to impulsive and destructive behaviours. For these reasons, crisis management is a crucial skill to develop, serving as a practice of self-care and compassion that supports survival and growth on the path to healing.

Identifying and naming a crisis can provide a sense of control, enabling appropriate responses and effective management of distress before it escalates. With a crisis management toolkit, emotional experiences become more manageable, reducing the feeling of being caught in an unending chaos. Understanding the unique signs of a crisis allows for selecting the most effective tools, helping to prevent further harm. This understanding also fosters self-compassion, replacing self-criticism with care during times of vulnerability.

Defining a Crisis

A crisis can be defined as a situation that is:

- Highly stressful
- Short-term in nature
- Accompanied by intense pressure to resolve immediately.

A crisis can be likened to a house fire—intensely traumatic but temporary. Immediate action is required to prevent further damage and destruction. Strong cravings align with this definition, causing significant physical and emotional stress, presenting as short-term experiences, and accompanied by a compelling urge to engage in addictive behaviour.

When to Use Crisis Management Skills

Crisis management skills should be employed when the following conditions are present:

- Severe emotional pain
- Urges to act impulsively on emotions.
- The actions considered would worsen the situation.
- Emotions threaten to overwhelm or are already overwhelming.
- The underlying issues cannot be resolved immediately.

These skills are designed specifically for situations of overwhelm, and not for managing all unpleasant emotional experiences. Overusing crisis management as a constant distraction or avoidance strategy can undermine the courage needed to progress on the healing journey.

The Crisis Gauge

A gauge such as the Subjective Units of Distress Scale (SUDS) can be used to determine when crisis management skills are necessary and to evaluate their effectiveness. This scale helps assess the level of distress, functioning like a thermometer to measure emotional intensity.

Figure 17 - The Subjective Units of Distress Scale (SUDS)

Subjective Units of Distress (SUDS)

01	Feeling calm, at ease. No distress, just totally relaxed.
02	Alert and awake, concentrating well. Feeling okay, neutral.
03	First awareness of tension, stress. Mild irritation; some anxiety, distress.
04	Some anxiety and distress; noticeable discomfort and irritation but it is tolerable.
05	Uncomfortable distress and discomfort; tolerable and not yet interfering with the ability to focus.
06	Distress is moderate to strong; it is interfering with the ability to focus and function.
07	Strong distress; interfering with ability to function. Emotional pain feels very uncomfortable.
08	Very distressed and uncomfortable; unable to concentrate; difficult to shift thoughts away from the distress.
09	Emotional distress feels extremely uncomfortable and intolerable.
10	The highest distress, anxiety, fear, or discomfort you have ever felt.

SUDS 7-10
Don't go it alone reach out to your Support System

According to the SUDS, entering the red zone (starting around 7) signals a crisis. At this level, functioning is impaired, and physical symptoms may indicate that emotional distress is taking over. Below 7, while distress may still be present, it is manageable. Crisis management techniques become essential when logical thinking becomes impaired and physical symptoms intensify.

The First Step: STOP!

The primary goal of crisis management is to reduce distress on the SUDS scale, restoring clear thinking and enabling choices that support health, wellbeing and healing. However, during a crisis, the logical thinking part of the brain may shut down, leaving the individual at the mercy of survival instincts. The first step in regaining control involves using the STOP technique:

Stop: Refrain from reacting immediately. Freeze and stay in place, whether standing, sitting, or lying down, as impaired judgment could influence immediate movement.

Take a step back: Mentally and physically, create distance from the situation. A physical step back can signal to the body and mind that control is being reasserted. Take several deep breaths, which are crucial in calming the body and restoring a sense of peace. The deep breaths can reduce the intensity of the crisis, facilitating more constructive responses.

Observe: Assess the surroundings, noting what is happening in the environment and the actions of others. Internally, identify current thoughts by naming them, e.g., "I am having the thought that...". This phrasing creates distance from the thought, offering perspective and enabling more mindful decision-making.

Proceed mindfully: Acknowledge the choice point: whether to act on impulses or take actions aligned with self-care and healing goals.

Preparing for a Crisis

During a crisis, intense urges can make it difficult to spontaneously think of alternative actions. Therefore, preparation in advance is highly recommended. Just as one might prepare for storm season with an emergency kit, preparing for emotional crises on the healing journey can be a compassionate and practical step. Establishing a crisis plan, including alternative actions, ensures that supportive strategies are readily available when needed, empowering you to act proactively rather than reactively.

Alternative Actions

Outlined below are various actions that can be taken instead of yielding to urges or impulses during a crisis. Experimentation may be necessary to determine which techniques are most effective:

Movement: Doing physical activity—dancing, running, punching, or jumping—can release anxiety and stimulate calming hormones. Intense exercise is particularly effective.

Keeping exercise equipment accessible, such as having running shoes at the door or a yoga mat readily available, can facilitate quick engagement.

Cold exposure: Placing the face in ice water can trigger a survival response, redirecting blood flow to essential organs and promoting effective thinking. Alternative quick options include using a cold, wet cloth stored in the freezer, or a ziplock bag of chilled water applied to the eyes.

Listening to music: Music has a powerful ability to heal and connect, offering comfort and inspiration. Creating a playlist of soothing or motivational songs can provide a sense of support during challenging moments.

Muscle tension exercises: Tensing muscles as a response to distress can paradoxically prompt relaxation. By exaggerating tension, the brain is signalled to initiate a relaxation response. This technique can be used discreetly, such as tensing and releasing muscle groups while breathing deeply.

Engaging the senses: Distracting from distress by focusing on the five senses can be grounding. For example, identifying five things to see, hear, smell, touch, and, if appropriate, taste can redirect focus away from overwhelming emotions.

Aromatherapy: Essential oils can directly influence the brain through olfactory pathways, helping to soothe or energise as needed. Lavender, known for its calming properties or uplifting scents like May Chang or Sweet Orange, can be used to break the cycle of crisis emotions.

Watching television: While not a long-term strategy, watching a distracting television show or movie can provide temporary relief from distress. It is a short-term fix and should not replace the development of skills to sit with and manage emotions.

Sleep: Going to bed can be a practical response when other strategies fail. Sleep offers a respite from distress, allowing emotions to subside naturally over time.

Establishing a set of reliable strategies, such as maintaining a playlist for crises or a specific physical activity, can create mental shortcuts that facilitate swift action during moments of distress. Preparing a personalised crisis kit and identifying supportive techniques can be one of the kindest and most empowering steps in the healing process, ensuring readiness to face the inevitable challenges with resilience and care.

Core Concepts

During healing, intense emotions or cravings can overwhelm and lead to impulsive actions. Crisis management is crucial for self-care and managing these moments.

A crisis is a highly stressful, short-term event needing immediate resolution, much like a house fire.

Crisis Management Steps (STOP Technique):
- Stop: Pause and avoid immediate reaction; stay in place.
- Take a step back: Mentally and physically distance yourself; take deep breaths to calm.
- Observe: Note surroundings, thoughts, and emotions to gain perspective.
- Proceed mindfully: Choose actions aligned with self-care rather than impulses.

Alternative Actions for Crisis Management:
- Movement: Physical activity releases anxiety.
- Cold exposure: Ice water reduce crisis intensity.
- Music: Play soothing or motivational songs.
- Muscle tension exercises to prompt relaxation.
- Engaging the senses to ground yourself.
- Watching television for temporary distraction.
- Sleep: Rest to allow emotions to settle naturally.

Preparing in advance with a crisis plan and identifying effective strategies can empower proactive responses during distress.

Having a personalised crisis toolkit fosters resilience and readiness for emotional challenges.

Essential Skill: Self-Compassion

"People are like stained-glass windows. They sparkle and shine when the sun is out, but when the darkness sets in, their true beauty is revealed only if there is a light from within." ~ Elisabeth Kubler-Ross

On some days, even while sober, the pressures of life can become overwhelming, overshadowing optimism and discipline. These are the times when the sky's beauty goes unnoticed, and the inner critic becomes louder. Between moments of sadness, there is often an effort to understand the underlying messages of these emotions. On such days, the practice of self-compassion becomes invaluable. For those who have lost friends and loved ones through addiction, it may be difficult to find a shoulder to cry on. Learning to soothe, care and love yourself then, is an essential skill. In my mind true healing is impossible without practicing self-compassion.

Several pivotal moments along the healing journey have bolstered the ability to navigate challenges, such as letting go of rigid expectations, seeking proactive support, and maintaining honesty about inner struggles. These actions are all grounded in the practice of self-compassion, which enables dealing with traumatic memories and present-day distressing emotions. Self-compassion facilitates the shift from mere acceptance to self-love and care, fostering independence and resilience. It serves as a guiding light, enabling personal growth and sharing one's spirit with the world. The power of self-compassion has been foundational in reaching a place of connection and sharing.

Understanding Self-Compassion

> *"Self-compassion is simply giving the same kindness to ourselves that we would give to others." ~ Christopher Germer*

At its core, self-compassion involves redirecting the kindness and care we usually extend to others towards ourselves. For instance, consider a friend struggling with alcoholism who, after a period of sobriety, experiences a relapse and expresses self-criticism and despair. The natural response might include:

- Offering comfort.
- Countering negative self-talk with positive reinforcement.
- Reminding the friend of past successes and the potential to learn from setbacks.

This response stems from knowing the friend's intrinsic worth and the desire to alleviate their suffering, guiding them to a place of hope and resilience.

However, this same compassion is often not extended inwardly. Personal setbacks may trigger a cycle of self-criticism and judgment, echoing negative external voices and reinforcing feelings of brokenness and inadequacy. This internal harshness contrasts sharply with the compassionate response given to others. It highlights the importance of practising self-compassion oneself.

"You've been criticising yourself for years, and it hasn't worked. Try approving of yourself and see what happens".
~Louise L. Hay

What if, instead of hating yourself, you treated yourself like a friend who was suffering? What if instead of coming into this situation with the intent to punish yourself, you entered with the purpose to practice self-compassion? I wonder what would happen.

The Elements of Self-Compassion

Kristen Neff outlines three core components of self-compassion:

1. **Mindful Awareness of Suffering**: Recognising one's pain without judgment or over-identification with negative emotions.
2. **Acknowledgement of Shared Humanity**: Understanding that suffering is a universal aspect of the human experience, connecting individuals rather than isolating them.

3. **Feelings and Actions of Compassion**: Responding to personal suffering with kindness and taking actions that nurture and support wellbeing.

Mindful Awareness of Suffering

Identifying personal distress can be more challenging than recognising it in others. Often, there is a tendency to dismiss personal suffering, urging oneself to "soldier on" without acknowledging the extent of the discomfort. This avoidance may serve as a protective mechanism but denies the opportunity to address the pain compassionately. Acknowledging that suffering exists is the first step towards seeking relief and healing.

Acknowledging Shared Humanity

This element emphasises the connection with the broader human experience. Recognising that suffering is not unique but part of a shared condition helps prevent becoming overly fixated on personal pain. This acknowledgment fosters a sense of community and access to collective wisdom and courage from others who are also navigating their challenges. It encourages moving beyond self-absorption and embracing a broader perspective.

Feelings and Actions of Compassion

The final step involves the courageous act of fully experiencing personal pain and responding with a desire to alleviate it. This process does not involve avoiding or repressing emotions but embracing them with care and supportive actions. Thich Nhat Hanh beautifully compares this process to the care shown to a distressed child.

"It's like a mother. When the baby is crying, she picks up the baby, and she holds the baby tenderly in her arms. Your pain, your anxiety is your baby. You have to take care of it. You have to go back to yourself, to recognise the suffering in you, embrace the suffering, and you get a relief" ~Thich Nhat Hanh.

Similarly, self-compassion involves tenderly holding one's pain, leading to relief and healing.

Misconceptions About Self-Compassion

There are many misconceptions about what self-compassion is. Some may see it as being soft, indulgent or condoning cruel behaviour. It is none of these things. Self-compassion is also not:

Dependent: Self-compassion is not contingent on external approval, specific actions, or perceived worthiness. It is a consistent presence that acknowledges the inherent value of every individual, regardless of circumstances.

Judgmental: While it acknowledges mistakes, self-compassion separates the person from their actions, encouraging responsibility and growth without harsh judgment.

Self-Indulgent: Self-compassion supports actions that sustain long-term wellbeing rather than providing immediate but detrimental gratification.

Self-Pity: Unlike self-pity, which fixates on personal suffering, self-compassion connects individual pain to the shared human condition, fostering resilience and communal strength.

A Short-Term Fix: Self-compassion goes beyond immediate comfort, guiding actions that nurture the present and future self. It encourages self-care practices that sustain emotional and physical wellbeing over time.

Practicing Self-Compassion

The transformative potential of self-compassion necessitates practice and commitment. Like any new behaviour, it requires time to become ingrained, especially when countering longstanding patterns of self-criticism, shame, and fear. As these unhelpful habits are unlearned, self-compassion cultivates new pathways for acceptance, resilience, and joy.

The most critical aspect of self-compassion is to begin the practice, embracing the present moment as an opportunity for growth.

For those seeking further resources on self-compassion, Dr. Kristin Neff's work provides valuable guidance. Her website, selfcompassion.org, offers a wealth of information and practical tools to support the development of self-compassion skills.

There are two simple self-compassion exercises that I would highly recommend. These are the:

1. Self-compassion break
2. Creation of a compassionate friend.

The Self-Compassion Break

The Self-Compassion Break is a quick, simple practice to cultivate self-kindness during stressful moments by addressing the three elements of self-compassion: mindfulness, common humanity, and self-kindness. Here's how:

- **Acknowledge your pain**. Say, "This is a moment of suffering," or something similar like "This hurts" or "This is stress."
- **Recognize shared humanity**. Remind yourself, "Suffering is part of life," or choose phrases like "I'm not alone" or "Others feel this way too."
- **Offer yourself kindness**. Place your hand on your heart and say, "May I be kind to myself." You can also set specific intentions like "May I forgive myself" or "May I be strong."

You can extend this practice by asking, "What do I need to hear right now to be kind to myself?" This technique can be practiced anytime to foster compassion and emotional resilience.

Creation of a Compassionate Friend

Sometimes it can be difficult to launch straight into showing compassion for yourself. However, there is an interim step you might like to try and this is conjuring a compassionate friend. In this exercise, you bring to mind someone you know who is:

- Wise. They have a range of tools and skills to calm emotional storms, and know just which one to use for the situation.
- Caring. This person displays kindness and warmth and is also committed to help you take responsibility for your own life and to be the best person you can be.
- Courageous. This person can face pain and suffering without being overwhelmed and establishes boundaries for the safety and wellbeing of themselves and others.

Then, during your moments of suffering, when you feel lost and alone, you can imagine your compassionate friend coming to sit beside you. You can imagine them holding you and loving you. Sometimes, all they may need to do is to be with you. At other times, when you are unsure about what your next step should be, you can always ask them for their advice.

"What would my compassionate friend do?"

Core Concepts

Healing from addiction can be overwhelming, with moments when self-compassion becomes essential, especially if external support is limited.

Self-compassion is crucial for dealing with trauma, distress, and setbacks, helping shift from acceptance to self-love, fostering independence and resilience.

Self-Compassion involves treating yourself with the same kindness you would extend to a friend.

Three Elements of Self-Compassion (Kristen Neff):
1. Mindful Awareness of Suffering: Recognising personal pain without judgment.
2. Acknowledgement of Shared Humanity: Understanding suffering is universal, creating connection rather than isolation.
3. Feelings and Actions of Compassion: Responding to personal suffering with kindness and supportive actions.

Self-Compassion is not self-indulgence, self-pity, or weakness; it's about maintaining boundaries, promoting accountability, and nurturing growth.

For further guidance, Dr. Kristin Neff's work on selfcompassion.org offers valuable resources and practical tools.

Conclusion

Knowledge ≠ Power

Knowledge + Action = Power

This principle underscores the essence of Addiction Healing Pathway: while gaining insights into addiction's complexities is crucial, true transformation occurs when this understanding is paired with intentional, compassionate action.

As explored in this book, *Understanding Addiction*, the path to recovery requires not only awareness of addiction's multifaceted nature but also the commitment to working progressively through the mental, emotional, and spiritual disconnections that have caused it.

The journey through understanding and healing from addiction is complex, deeply personal, and often fraught with challenges. So, here are some key points to take with you:

Addiction is a Symptom: Rather than being the core problem, addiction often serves as a coping mechanism for deeper psychological or emotional pain. Understanding this can shift the focus from mere symptom management to addressing the root causes of distress.

The Cause of Addiction: The root cause of addiction is a disconnect with your spirit. This fundamental issue has set off a whole war within you, and the conflict has created many casualties. It has resulted in you feeling faulty, unworthy and led you to undertake acts of self-harm. Reuniting with your spirit will not be easy, but it will bring a sustainable sense of passion and peace that can rival the pleasure gained from the addictive substances or behaviours.

The Addiction Healing Pathway: This model offers a simple and structured guide not only to get started on your healing journey, but to see how you are progressing along the way. You can use the Addiction Healing Pathway to determine what areas of your healing are working well, and where more work is required to bring them back into a healthy balance. It is a simple and useful reminder about the holistic elements of healing - the body, mind, emotions, environment and spirit.

Healing is a Process of Moving from Force to Power: Addiction is filled with force emotions, including shame, guilt, fear and anger. All of these are valid responses to a range of troubling life experiences and a consequence of being separated from your spirit. However, with awareness, and with The Addiction Healing Pathway, one has the ability to progress past these life-destroying emotions and move towards those that bring life, love and deep fulfilment. With courage we can move beyond those things that are keeping us stuck and hear the call of our spirit.

Combining Scientific and Spiritual Approaches: Effective healing from addiction requires integrating scientific and spiritual elements. While scientific approaches provide essential insights into the neurological, psychological, and behavioural aspects of addiction, spiritual practices can address the deeper emotional and existential voids often at the heart of addictive behaviours. A holistic approach acknowledges the importance of evidence-based treatments, such as medical intervention and therapy, alongside spiritual practices like mindfulness, meditation, and self-compassion.

Essential Skills - Crisis Management and Self-Compassion: If you are a person struggling with addiction or are someone caring for a loved one, there are two skills that are always beneficial to build. The first is Crisis Management, which will help you deal with emotional distress in constructive ways. The second is Self-Compassion which will help you move away from the Force emotions of Shame and Anger and find the courage needed to take actions grounded in love.

A Reminder to Reach Out for Help:

If you or someone you care about is struggling with addiction, remember that help is available. Seeking assistance is a courageous and vital step toward healing. Numerous organisations and professionals are dedicated to supporting individuals through their healing journey. Whether through medical professionals, support groups, or community services, reaching out can provide the guidance and encouragement needed to move forward.

Though challenging, your journey toward healing is entirely possible with the right support and resources. Your strength in seeking help can pave the way for a healthier, more fulfilling life for yourself and those you care about.

And remember:

You are worthy of health and happiness!

Who To Call

If you are experiencing any distressing feelings and would like someone to talk these through with, please contact the following organisations. They would love to help.

Lifeline Australia

www.lifeline.org.au

13 11 14

Lifeline Australia provides a free, confidential and anonymous, 24-hour telephone counselling service for adults needing emotional support. Lifeline Australia also has a range of information and resources available from their website, about providing care in times of crisis.

The Salvation Army

www.salvationarmy.org.au

13 SALVOS (13 72 58)

One of Australia's largest providers of alcohol and other drugs treatment services. They provide hope, compassion and dignity to support you as you overcome your challenges.

Beyond Blue

www.beyondblue.org.au

1300 22 4636

Beyond Blue is a national organisation that has a range of information and resources associated with depression and anxiety. The Support Service runs 24 hours a day, seven days a week. All calls are one-on-one with a trained mental health professional and completely confidential.

Black Dog Institute

www.blackdoginstitute.org.au

The Black Dog Institute provides a 24-hour free mobile phone/computer-based programme to assist those with mild to moderate depression, anxiety and stress.

References

[1] Gowing, L. R., Ali, R. L., Allsop, S., Marsden, J., Turf, E. E., West, R., & Witton, J. (2015). Global statistics on addictive behaviours: 2014 status report. Addiction, 110(6), 904–919. https://doi.org/10.1111/add.12899

[2] National Institute on Drug Abuse. (2020, April 13). What is the scope of prescription drug misuse? Retrieved from https://www.drugabuse.gov/publications/research-reports/misuse-prescription-drugs/what-scope-prescription-drug-misuse

[3] Shannon, M. (2016, September 14). Why is Internet Addiction Growing in Asia? The Cabin Chiang Mai. https://www.thecabinchiangmai.com/blog/why-is-internet-addiction-growing-in-asia/

[4] Lexico.Com. https://www.lexico.com/definition/addicted

[5] America, M. I. (2023, March 3). The power of Addiction and the addiction to power | Gabor Maté, MD - Mad in America. Mad in America. https://www.madinamerica.com/2022/03/the-power-of-addiction-and-the-addiction-to-power-gabor-mate-md/

[6] Lexico.Com. https://www.lexico.com/definition/choice

[7] Dr. Kevin McCauley – Pleasure Unwoven: Addiction Education Society. (n.d.). Retrieved from https://addictioneducationsociety.org/dr-kevin-mccauley-pleasure-unwoven/

[8] Addiction Is a Disease of Free Will: Addiction Education Society. (n.d.). Retrieved January 15, 2021, from

https://addictioneducationsociety.org/addiction-is-a-disease-of-free-will/

[9] Lexico.Com. https://www.lexico.com/definition/disease

[10] Mental disorders. (2019, November 28). WHO | World Health Organization. https://www.who.int/news-room/fact-sheets/detail/mental-disorders

[11] Hasin, D. S., O'Brien, C. P., Auriacombe, M., Borges, G., Bucholz, K., Budney, A., Compton, W. M., Crowley, T., Ling, W., Petry, N. M., Schuckit, M., & Grant, B. F. (2013). DSM-5 criteria for substance use disorders: recommendations and rationale. The American journal of psychiatry, 170(8), 834–851. https://doi.org/10.1176/appi.ajp.2013.12060782

[12] Lewis, M. (2015). The biology of desire: Why addiction is not a disease. Scribe Publications.

[13] Why addiction isn't a disease but instead the result of 'deep learning' | NDARC - National drug and alcohol research centre. (n.d.). National Drug and Alcohol Research Centre (NDARC). https://ndarc.med.unsw.edu.au/blog/why-addiction-isnt-disease-instead-result-deep-learning

[14] Lexico.Com. https://www.lexico.com/definition/symptom

[15] Berger, W. (2016). A More Beautiful Question: The Power of Inquiry to Spark Breakthrough Ideas (Reprint ed.). Bloomsbury USA.

[16] Ph.D., Hollis. J. (2020). Living Between Worlds: Finding Personal Resilience in Changing Times. Sounds True.

[17] PhD, Lewis, M. (2016). The Biology of Desire: Why Addiction Is Not a Disease. PublicAffairs

[18] America, M. I. (2023, March 3). The power of Addiction and the addiction to power | Gabor Maté, MD - Mad in America. Mad in America.

https://www.madinamerica.com/2022/03/the-power-of-addiction-and-the-addiction-to-power-gabor-mate-md/

[19] https://centerhealthyminds.org/

[20] Bennet, B & Green, S. Our Voices: Aboriginal Social Work. (2019). Red Globe Press.

[21] Ingerman, S. (2015). Walking in Light: The Everyday Empowerment of a Shamanic Life (First PB Edition, First Printing ed.). Sounds True.

[22] Rinpoche, T. W., & Turner, P. (2015). The True Source of Healing: How the Ancient Tibetan Practice of Soul Retrieval Can Transform and Enrich Your Life. Hay House Inc.

[23] Griffith, J., & Prosen, H. (2016). FREEDOM: The End Of The Human Condition (2nd ed.). WTM Publishing and Communications.

[24] Lexico.Com. https://www.lexico.com/definition/stigma

[25] https://www.rethinkaddiction.org.au

[26] https://www.sbs.com.au/programs/addicted-australia

[27] Ingerman, S. (2015). Walking in Light: The Everyday Empowerment of a Shamanic Life (First PB Edition, First Printing ed.). Sounds True.

[28] Rehabilitation Drugs - What Treatment Drugs Are Used to Assist in Rehab? (2020, March 9). American Addiction Centers. https://americanaddictioncenters.org/addiction-medications

[29] Addiction withdrawal symptoms. (n.d.). Healthdirect. Retrieved April 9, 2021, from https://www.healthdirect.gov.au/addiction-withdrawal-symptoms

[30] Makin, S., 2020. Deep Sleep Gives Your Brain A Deep Clean. [online] Scientific American. Available at: <https://www.scientificamerican.com/article/deep-sleep-gives-your-brain-a-deep-clean1/> [Accessed 20 August 2020].

[31] McGonigal, K. (2021). The Joy of Movement: How exercise helps us find happiness, hope, connection, and courage. Avery.

[32] Developed by Dr Russ Harris and published in the following book: Harris, R., 2008. The Happiness Trap. Shambala Press.

[33] Dethmer, J., Chapman, D Leadership. and Klemp, K., n.d. The 15 Commitments Of Conscious.

[34] Dethmer, J., Chapman, D Leadership. and Klemp, K., n.d. The 15 Commitments Of Conscious.

[35] Taylor, J. B. (2006). My stroke of insight: A brain scientist's personal journey. New York, NY: Penguin Books.

[36] Hawkins, D. (2002). Power vs. force. Carlsbad, Calif.: Hay House.

[37] https://www.lexico.com/definition/courage

[38] Harris, R., 2011. The Confidence Gap. Boston: Trumpeter

[39] Purifying Negative Karma. (n.d.). Https://Thubtenchodron.Org. https://thubtenchodron.org/1992/08/purify-negative-karma/

[40] The Top Five Regrets of the Dying: A Life Transformed by the Dearly Departing, Bronnie Ware, 2012, Hay House Inc.

[41] Tenzin Wangyal Rinpoche, The True Source of Healing, Hay House, 2015

[42] A. Van Den Broeck, B. Schreurs, K. Proost, A. Vanderstukken, M. Vansteenkiste, I want to be a billionaire:

How do extrinsic and intrinsic values influence youngsters' wellbeing? Ann. Am. Acad. Pol. Soc. Sci. 682, 204–219 (2019).

[43] Macy, J., & Johnstone, C. (2012). Active Hope: How to Face the Mess We're in without Going Crazy (58069th ed.). New World Library.

[44] Fowler, J. and Christakis, N., 2008. Dynamic spread of happiness in a large social network: longitudinal analysis over 20 years in the Framingham Heart Study. BMJ, 337(dec04 2), pp.a2338-a2338.

[45] Huffingtonpost.com.au. 2020. Available at: <https://www.huffingtonpost.com.au/entry/qualities-of-real-friends_n_5709821> [Accessed 16 August 2020]

P.S.

About the author

About the Understanding Series

Read on

Find out about the next book

Meet Belinda Tobin

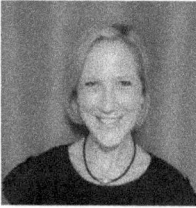

Belinda Tobin is a researcher, author, producer, and avid explorer of the human experience with all its challenges and complexities. Her works span fiction, non-fiction, poetry, tv series and film. However, they all share a common purpose, to foster a more conscious, compassionate and connected future.

Find out more about Belinda and her projects at www.belindatobin.com.

About the Understanding Series

"The highest form of ignorance is when you reject something you don't know anything about." — Wayne Dyer

Understanding Press was founded with a simple yet profound mission: to help each of us step into our power through knowledge and to pave the way for wise action.

The Understanding Series is the first project for Understanding Press. It provides clear and concise information about some of the most fundamental issues and pressing problems of our time. Here are the current titles in The Understanding Series.

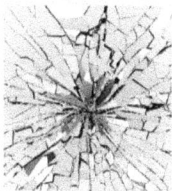

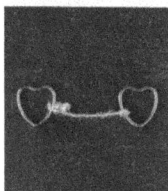

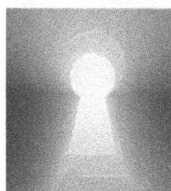

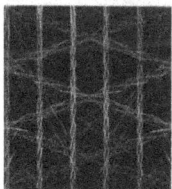

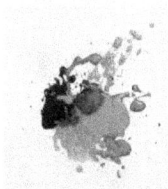

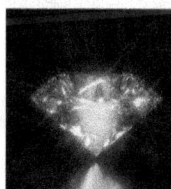

Read On- Understanding Monogamy

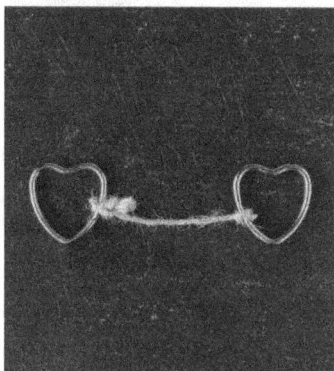

A pathway to conscious and compassionate connections.

Our intimate relationships are in a state of flux. Marriage, once considered a sacred institution, is increasingly overlooked, while divorce is a common feature of family life. Online, millions tune in to see cheaters exposed, and more people are exploring alternative arrangements like open marriages and polyamory. These trends suggest that monogamy, as traditionally practised, may no longer align with the needs of our modern, secular society—or that our current model is fundamentally flawed.

Understanding Monogamy explores the idea that while monogamy is not natural, it has become the norm, creating a moral dilemma for individuals and society. Science has shown that humans are not inherently suited for lifelong, exclusive partnerships. Yet, monogamy persists, and rejecting it without understanding its roots only replicates the conflicts it creates. This book delves into how monogamy became the default relationship model and exposes the myths that distort our expectations of it.

While societal change may continue to challenge monogamy, it remains the gold standard for many. To reduce the suffering caused by unmet expectations, Understanding Monogamy encourages readers to examine their own beliefs about love and sex and how these shape their experiences in relationships. By developing a deeper understanding of these dynamics, individuals can navigate coupledom with greater awareness and authenticity.

Understanding Monogamy is an essential guide for anyone considering a sexually exclusive relationship, struggling within one, or exploring alternatives. It provides valuable insights and practical guidance, helping readers make conscious, compassionate choices in their pursuit of love. Because everyone deserves a relationship that is true to who they are and filled with love.

Read On- Understanding Violence

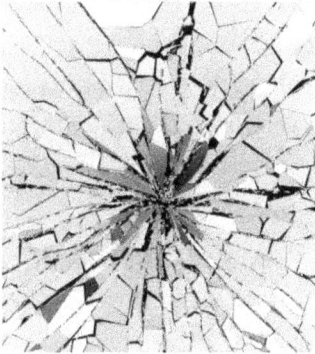

"Peace cannot be kept by force; it can only be achieved by understanding." – Albert Einstein.

Understanding Violence is a heartfelt exploration born from the author's continued distress at the family and domestic violence crisis that has been continuing for decades. To solve the problem of violence, we must first fully understand it, not just one part, but its totality. This book goes beyond the headlines, delving into the varied and often hidden ways violence manifests in our society—from the overt to the subtle, from the physical to the psychological. It shows family violence as one traumatic symptom of a much larger disease. Reducing violence in society then is not just about pointing fingers at "bad people"; it's about understanding the culture that allows violence to thrive and recognising that we all play a role in its perpetuation.

Drawing from research, personal reflections, and expert insights, the author emphasises that understanding is the first crucial step toward change. By calling out violence in all its forms and unpacking the beliefs, emotions, and systemic issues that underpin violent behaviours, Understanding Violence invites readers to reflect on their own actions and the world around them. It challenges us to look honestly at how violence infiltrates our everyday lives, whether through media, politics, entertainment or unexamined attitudes.

This book is for anyone who believes in a more compassionate, peaceful world. Whether you're a policymaker, a community leader, or someone seeking to make a difference in your own life, Understanding Violence offers insights to help break the cycle of harm at the source. By fostering a deeper understanding, we can all contribute to meaningful change—starting with ourselves.

www.ingramcontent.com/pod-product-compliance
Lightning Source LLC
Chambersburg PA
CBHW052123270326
41930CB00012B/2741

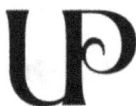

UNDERSTANDING PRESS

For more titles, go to:

www.heart-led.pub/understanding-press